Breathing

Breathing

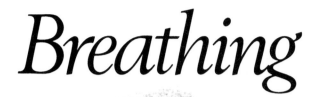

EXPANDING
your
POWER & ENERGY

Michael Sky

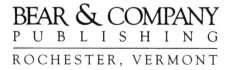

BEAR & COMPANY
PUBLISHING
ROCHESTER, VERMONT

LIBRARY OF CONGRESS CATALOGING-IN-PUBLICATION DATA
Sky, Michael, 1951-
Breathing : expanding your power & energy / by Michael Sky.
p.   cm.
ISBN 0-939680-82-3
1. Breathing exercises. I. Title.
RA782.S585 1990
613'.192—dc20   90-840
                                                                   CIP

Bear & Company, Inc.
Rochester, Vermont
Bear & Company is a division of Inner Traditions International
www.InnerTraditions.com

Cover illustration: Catherine Kenward © 1986
Author photo: Marie Favorito © 1988
Interior illustration: Angela C. Werneke
Cover & interior design: Angela C. Werneke
Editing: Barbara Doern Drew
Typography: Casa Sin Nombre, Ltd.
Printed in the United States

9

*This is for my parents
and for the gift of breath.*

Special Notice to the Reader

This book describes a breathing practice ("circular breathing") that can be greatly empowering and that is especially suited for self-healing. Fifteen years of working with circular breathing—personally and professionally—has led the author to conclude that for all its power, it is an inherently safe practice. Nonetheless, it sometimes initiates a process that can be physically and/or emotionally intense and quite upsetting. Thus, the reader should approach circular breathing with gentle caution. Neither the author nor the publisher can assure that any of the practices described in this book will be perfectly safe in all instances.

Contents

Acknowledgments 11

Preface 13

I. Simple Human Alchemy 21

II. The Conscious Embodiment of Spirit 27

III. Energy in Motion 33

IV. The Dynamics of Response 41

V. The Formation of Primary Patterns 47

VI. Pain, Separation & the Habits of a Lifetime 53

VII. Lessons in Breath 61

VIII. The Circle of Breath 69

IX. Partners in Breath 75

X. Rapture, Excitement & the Lessons of Sleep 83

XI. The Continuing Process of Resolution 93

XII. Sexual Energy & the Energetic Embrace 101

XIII. Sexual Communion 111

XIV. The Holy Breath 121

Appendix A: Conscious Breathing Patterns 129

Appendix B: Kundalini Crisis & Spiritual Emergency 139

Appendix C: The Breath We Share 141

Notes 143

Permissions 147

About the Author 149

Acknowledgments

With gratitude:

to Leonard Orr for the baptism of water and air and
all that has followed;

to Da Free John—though we've never met, his crazy
wisdom permeates my life and writing;

to everyone at Bear for another easy dance;

to Tina Rose and Sue Ann Fazio for early readings and
good advice;

to Lee and Susan and happy breathing Benjamin;

to all my friends and students—to every willing body
I've ever sat with in patient silence, sharing breath;

and to Penny, fellow mariner through storm and
calm—are they not all the seas of God?

Preface

In his utopian fiction, *Island*, author Aldous Huxley created a world in which trained parrots were always hovering about, saying, "Be here now, boys, be here now," as a constant reminder to the natives to stay in the present moment.

If I could give a parrot with each copy of *Breathing*, it would sit on the reader's shoulder, whispering gently, "Breathing, breathing, breathing, breathing. . . " For this is a book to be breathed, even as it is read. And it is a book that will be best understood, and rendered effective, through the direct, conscious participation of the reader, via the breath.

Throughout the book there are simple breathing exercises, or explorations, that are intended to be experienced *as you read*. An important message of *Breathing* is that we can become conscious of our breath during any and all of the activities of our daily lives and that it is greatly empowering to do so.

Thus, you can become conscious of your breath in this moment—you can *feel* the inward and outward flows of life—while continuing to read these words, and while reading through to the end of the page and through to the end of the book. Your understanding of the breath will be enhanced through such conscious reading/breathing. Even more, the lessons of the book will be *embodied*. With practice, we can become increasingly conscious of the breath—from moment to moment to moment—becoming increasingly conscious, and inspired, as human "breathings."

My own journey into the power of breath began early in life. I can remember being small enough to crawl inside a pillowcase, curling into a fetal position, and then taking a deep breath and holding it for as long as possible. I now understand that I was performing a basic exercise found in the disciplines of Chinese *chi kung* ("manipulation of vital energy") and yogic *pranayama* ("expansion of vital energy"), and that I was purposefully using my breath to energize and empower myself.

I believe that I was healing myself—that I was causing positive changes that have enabled me to grow into the person I am today—though I can only wonder how I knew to take such steps. Furthermore, I strongly suspect that all children engage in "advanced" breathing/healing practices, only to forget them as the habits of age literally take the breath away.

When I reached college, I began searching for ways to remember breathing, beginning with the practice of yoga and *pranayama*. I found that while I had little patience for sitting in passive silence, I became totally committed to what I have come to think of as active breathing meditations.

I would walk for miles, timing my inhale and exhale to the cadence of my steps. I would sit in class breathing in through the right nostril and out through the left, feeling for the subtle effects while noticing that my attention to the teacher actually improved. Sitting in traffic, I would take a deep breath, holding it in, while relaxing the muscles of my body and releasing the pressures of the day. Gradually, such conscious breathing became a regular part of my life, a continuous stream of active awareness that seemed to enhance everything I was doing.

In 1975, my experience of the breath was powerfully expanded when I met Leonard Orr and was "rebirthed" for the first time. The practice of rebirthing grew out of Leonard's insight that we learn to breathe at birth and that our early lessons are often poorly handled, with tragic results.

The rebirthing process in those days involved floating in a hot tub and breathing through a snorkel until one's "birth trauma" was remembered and resolved, and new patterns were established. The process could be explosively intense. Within minutes of beginning my first rebirthing, my entire body cramped into the most incredible pain I have ever experienced. Slowly the pain subsided, leaving an ecstatic, tingling glow in its wake. I remember lying there thinking *I am a body, I am breathing*, over and over and over again, as if it were a startling new insight. Indeed it was, and one that has since inspired my every waking moment.

In the ensuing years, the rebirthing process—which I now call "circular breathing," to de-emphasize the importance of remembering birth—has been the central focus of my life. I have explored the practice with hundreds of friends and students, individually and in groups. I have been honored to witness, time and again, the precious moment of rebirth. I am forever impressed with the power of conscious circular breathing as a tool for personal transformation, as well as with its inherent safety and simplicity.

My purpose in writing has been to thoroughly describe the dynamics of conscious breathing, while providing the details of a regular breathing practice. I believe that any reader who conscientiously applies the principles in *Breathing* will experience a wondrous expansion of vital energy, an unending source of personal power, and a magically heightened capacity for joy. This is, at last, simple human alchemy, a fusion of the heart; we are learning to breathe spirit into flesh.

May your every breath bring peace and joy.
May all beings breathe free and flourish.

Breathing

Sail forth—steer for the deep waters only,
Reckless O soul, exploring, I with thee,
    and thou with me,
For we are bound where mariner has not yet
    dared to go,
And we will risk the ship, ourselves and all.

O brave soul!
O farther farther sail!
O daring joy, but safe! are they not all
    the seas of God?
O farther, farther, farther sail!

Walt Whitman[1]

Begin by paying attention
  to your next few breaths.
Even as you continue to read these words,
  also notice that you are breathing
    and that it is easy to read and to breathe
    and to be aware of breath,
    all in the same moment.
Pay attention to the quality of each inhale.
Even as you read, notice the feelings and
  sensations of breath flowing into your body.
Feel the places in your torso that move
  or do not move with each inhalation.
Pay attention to the quality of each exhale.
Even as you read, notice the feelings and
  sensations of breath flowing from your body.
Feel the places in your torso that move
  or do not move with each exhalation.
Now return to the top of this page
  and read through again,
    paying close attention to the ebb and flow
    of each breath, even as you are paying
    close attention to the sound and meaning
    of each word, and for a minute or so,
    simply pay attention to yourself breathing,
  as your eyes softly close . . .

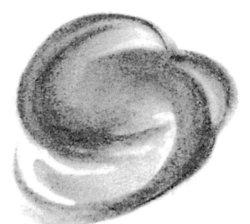

❋ I ❋
Simple Human Alchemy

It is so easy to take breathing for granted. Breath is a fully automatic process, beginning at birth and continuing without interruption until the day we die. More to the point, it can be a fully *unconscious* process — there is no need to attend consciously in any way one's breathing. Just as we can expect to breathe quite adequately while sleeping each night, so can we expect our breathing to continue without ever actually doing it. It is the nature of breath that it will continue through the deepest and most unconscious of human sleep.

Of course, our hearts also beat continuously without any conscious effort, and we digest our food without actually doing anything about it. From moment to moment throughout our lives, there are a thousand and one vital processes occurring in our bodies, of which we are generally unaware and uninformed. This is part of the wonderful design of living creatures: most of the workings of the body are driven by unconscious intelligence, so that conscious awareness is freed for other pursuits.

With the breath, however, we discover something of great importance. While breathing can well be a completely unconscious process, it also can quite easily become a conscious, intentional practice. That is, while it is critical that respiration, along with most of our bodily processes, be a continuously—and thus unconsciously—driven function, it is also possible to consciously influence and control the flow of breath. This unique quality of the breath—that it can be both conscious and unconscious—makes it a link between the conscious and unconscious aspects of our being.

You can stop your breathing now for several moments, if you want to. You can resume breathing deeply now, if you want to. You can fill your lungs completely with breath, or breathe very lightly, or let the air out in a gentle sigh, or blow it out in a strong wind, all because you want to—it is easily within your conscious control. It is really quite a simple matter to bring consciousness to the act of breathing.

It is the premise of this book, and of the many "teachings of the breath" that our world has known, that bringing consciousness to the act of breathing is of great physical, mental, emotional, and spiritual benefit to the human individual. And while there are many highly complex and often difficult ways to practice "bringing consciousness to the act of breathing," there are also many ways in which such practice can be simple, safe, and immediately accessible to all people.

Ultimately, in any moment that we are even slightly aware of the movement of breath within us, then we are more conscious as individuals and more directly involved in the integrated functions of body, mind, and spirit. Conscious breathing encourages the expansion of consciousness throughout the human organism and beyond: to inhale consciously is to positively excite and expand the whole environment of which one is a part; to exhale consciously is to support the relaxation of all surrounding and connecting energies. Truly, every moment of conscious breath is an inspired co-creation with life itself.

There should be no dead breath, no small chemistry, but intentional and full use of breathing as a feeling instrument in the actual and present ingestion, translation, and transfer of Life-Energy.

Da Free John[2]

The purpose of conscious breathing is not primarily the movement of air, but the movement of energy. If you do a relaxed, connected breathing cycle for a few minutes, you will begin to experience dynamic energy flows within your body. These energy flows are the merging of spirit and matter.

Leonard Orr[3]

Breathe deeply and gently through every cell of the body, laugh happily, and release the head of all worries and anxieties; and finally, breathe in the blessing of love, hope, and immortality that is flowing in the air, and you will understand the meaning of human breath.

Pundit Acharya[4]

Breathe in fully, and now hold the breath in.
Read to the bottom of this page,
  while continuing to hold your breath.
Do this without straining or struggling;
  if at any moment this begins to feel
    difficult, or stressful, or dizzying,
    then let the breath go, and start over again.
Allow your belly to be relaxed, loose, full,
  and round with breath.
Let your shoulders be relaxed and loose—
  sinking down rather than tensing up.
Notice any changes throughout your
  whole body and mind; pay attention to any
  and all feelings or sensations.
Do this for as long as it is easy to do so,
  retaining the breath, without stressing
  or straining.
When it is time to let go,
  release the breath calmly and
  quietly and smoothly.
Now repeat this process three times:
  breathing deeply, and then
    holding the breath for as long as possible,
    staying loose and relaxed,
    and then releasing the breath
    in a calm, quiet stream,
  as your eyes softly close . . .

✳ II ✳

The Conscious Embodiment of Spirit

An understanding of the full promise and power of the breath requires an understanding of the subtle aspects of the human organism. The strictly material explanations of living things that have so dominated the past three hundred years of Western thought have generated much that is good, certainly. But they have also steered around, or flatly discounted, a fundamental characteristic of all living systems.

Amoebas, whales, worms, and human beings all share, with all living creatures, one vital attribute: their physical forms are permeated with a subtle vibratory essence, called *energy*. This energy flows in regular currents within the physical body, and extends as radiant fields throughout the body and into the surrounding environment.[5] It is similar in quality and effect to electricity, magnetism, gravity, and nuclear force, while being different from all of these. Though difficult to grasp scientifically, this energy is easily experienced. With continued experience, one eventually comes to understand that energy is the essence of the body, mind, and spirit, and that it is the key to the healthy integration of human life.

Even without scientific substantiation, most people are well aware of the flow of energy in their lives. We talk of "having a lot of energy" or of "feeling low on energy"; of "moving forward with a full head of steam" or of "feeling like the fires have gone out." We know what it is to have sexual energy and mental energy. We can feel when a moment has a strong emotional "charge." We easily recognize the radiant glow of love and the powerful aura of good health. We understand well that *every-thing* that moves in our world is moved by some form of energy.

Furthermore, we understand that all matter in the universe is comprised of energy, as so elegantly expressed in Einstein's equation $E=mc^2$. We know that energy and matter are inter-convertible, that all matter is essentially frozen or crystallized energy, and that all matter is in the process of slowly or rapidly transforming into energy. We have spent a great deal of time and intellectual effort developing ways to more efficiently and use-fully control this movement of matter into energy—beginning with our first wood fires and culminating in our more recent nuclear reactions.

We understand very little, however, about the other half of the equation: the transformation of energy into mass. We do know that plants, for instance, take the energy of light (along with the more material aspects of earth, water, and air) and, through the process called photosynthesis, somehow convert that energy into material form. We still think of the creation of human bodies, though, strictly in terms of "building blocks": it is presumed that our material forms grow entirely out of the material constituents of food, water, air, and the genetic gifts of our parents. While we are beginning to see that "bad energies" (that is, radiation, unfiltered sunlight, radon, and excessive electromagnetism) can create pathological flesh, we are hardly even looking for the ways in which human bodies are the direct manifestation of energy into matter.

Every cell of the human body is, at its core, an atomic reactor of the most exquisite design that is continuously engaged in the conversion of matter into energy *and* energy into matter. The material constituents of this dual conversion process are carried to the heart of each cell via physical systems that are well understood by Western science; however, free-flowing universal energy is carried to the heart of each of cell as well by a subtle circulatory system that Western science has yet to describe.

Our breath is the living mechanism that drives this subtle circulatory system. *The primary way in which humans convert energy into physical form is through the breath.* With every breath we take, we are gathering and transforming the raw material of our bodies and minds.

Breathing energy into flesh begins in purely quantitative terms: the air that we breathe is replete with the energy of life, and it is our most direct and abundant source of "energy becoming mass." The more deeply and continuously we breathe, the more energy we gather, and the more possibilities for physical and mental transformation we enable.

There are also vital qualitative aspects to our breath: the degree of consciousness that we bring to our breathing determines the nature of our physical and mental manifestations. It is through breathing that energy gathers, circulates, and radiates throughout the many aspects of our being. The rate, rhythm, depth, intensity, physical manner, and mental attention of each breath contribute precisely to the movement and embodiment of energy within our lives.

Inspire: [L. *inspirare* < *in-* in + *spirare-* breath, courage, vigor, the soul, life] 1. to breathe 2. to infuse life into by breathing 3. to have an animating effect upon 4. to cause, guide, communicate, or motivate as by divine or supernatural influence.

Webster's New World Dictionary

And the Lord God formed man of the dust of the ground, and breathed into his nostrils the breath of life; and man became a living soul.

Genesis 2:7, King James Bible

Our breathing is the fragile vessel that carries us from birth to death.

Dr. Frederick Leboyer[6]

Breathe as lightly, and as quietly, as possible.
Even as you continue reading,
  breathe long, slow breaths,
    in and out through your nose,
      while imagining that just below
        your nostrils is a tray covered with ashes,
        and you must breathe ever so lightly,
        and ever so softly,
          not making even the slightest ripple of wind,
          nor the slightest vibration of sound,
      so that you will not disturb the ashes.
Let your body be loose and relaxed,
  for the slightest tension anywhere
    might disturb the ashes.
Let your mind be still, your thoughts quiet,
  for the slightest mental agitation
    might disturb the ashes.
For the next minute or so,
  continue breathing long, slowly, and
    ever so quietly, creating no disturbances,
      generating only peace,
      as your eyes softly close . . .

✳ III ✳

Energy in Motion

For the perfectly healthy, idealized human, energy would flow unimpeded from cell to cell and radiate without interference in overlapping, and interrelated, fields. This perfect movement of energy would nourish the body and guide its many processes; would uplift, enlighten, and continuously inspire the mind; and would radiate outward, as love, into intimate connection with the surrounding world. Such a rare and fortunate person would *feel good*, all of the time.

For the rest of us, the movement of energy is a far more tenuous affair. As we grow, we invariably develop patterns of tense and contracted energy, patterns that impair the free flow and perfect radiance of energy throughout all levels of our being. Our body cells become energy starved and suffer greatly. Our bodily functions are hampered and diminished. Our minds are likewise energy starved, and we experience excess mental stress and anxiety, leading to negativity and neurosis. We come to feel disconnected from others and from our environment. Typically, we *feel bad* much of the time, or, more tragically, *we lose the capacity to feel at all.*

With careful observation, it becomes apparent that those who *feel* life the most and have the greatest capacity for pleasure also have the most vital experience of energy; that feelings and energy are closely related, if not synonymous; and that *feeling good*—the highest priority of most all people, if not of their philosophies and religious systems—is a direct function of strong and vigorous energy.

Our feeling nature (what some have called our "emotional body") is our moment-to-moment experience of the movement of energy within our lives. To have a feeling is to be immediately aware of energy changing into mass and/or mass changing into energy; that is, to feel—whether fear, sadness, anger, excitement, happiness, joy—is to be aware of energy in motion and transformation through the various levels of self. Our feelings are comprised of energy, and they function as a fluid, moving interface between body, mind, spirit, and environment. If we are to be fully realized as human beings, then we must *feel* life, deeply, at all times.

Feelings arise as energetic balances to the events of our lives, allowing us to move through life with the greatest possibilities for success. Something happens, and we then feel a certain way. The feeling is a tangible movement of personal energy, giving us the substance of a healthy response. The feeling may be the energy of action or of emotional expression or of communication or of strong, willful resolve for the future. It may be the energy of deep thought, leading to a change of mind, or of deep

soul searching, leading to a change of heart. Feelings are a necessary condition of being fully alive, and they carry the raw material of effective response and meaningful change.

When we experience a threat to our well-being, we immediately generate energy to meet the threat, and we feel fright-
ened. The sensation of fear is the movement of energy needed
to resolve the threatening event. It is the substance of our
response—of fight or flight or transformational growth—and
the more we feel it, the more intelligent and balanced our
response will be.

When we experience the loss of a loved one or a cherished
dream, we immediately generate energy to address the loss, and
we feel sorrow. The sensation of sadness is the movement of
energy needed to resolve our hurt. It is the substance of our
response, allowing us to complete our relationship with the lost
one. The more we allow ourselves to feel our sorrows, the more
healing our responses will be, and the more compassionate we
will become for others facing similar losses.

When we experience interference with an important intention, we immediately generate strong energy to deal with the
barrier, and we likely feel angry. The sensation of anger is the
movement of energy needed to in some way overcome the barrier. It is the substance of our response—the energy of resolute
action, or of fresh insight into the problem, or of a positive,
active acceptance of the barrier. The more we allow ourselves to
feel our anger, the more successful we will be.

So it is with all human feelings: our emotions are forever
arising as energetic balances to the events of our lives. Unfortunately, if we are not trained or educated in such an awareness
of our feelings, and if we are in fact taught (formally and

indirectly) to resist the healthy movement of feeling/energy, then this essentially human, living response becomes perverted, resulting in serious and profound difficulties.

As an example, when we experience an intensely traumatizing event, our immediate and proper response is to contract on all levels—physical, mental, and especially energetic/emotional—from the source of the trauma. This contraction from a painful event can be witnessed in all living creatures; it is a natural, living mechanism and an important survival strategy.

In the same moment that we are contracting *away* from the event, we will also be generating strong currents of energy to empower us in our response *to* the event. This great influx of energy is held under intense contraction and within the mental context of "I don't want this!" All of this feels terrible. It is this overall energetic response, all occurring quite naturally in the moment of severe trauma, that we call a negative emotional experience.

If we do not experience the full resolution of such traumas, we obviously come to resist our negative emotions, a resistance that only adds to their negative impact. More importantly, when we fail to resolve traumatic events, they remain, in the form of contracted energy, a part of our continuing experience. During the event, we energetically contract; unless we release and resolve such a contraction, it will remain as a tangible wound or scar or disruptive pattern in our emotional body, which in turn can lead to mental neurosis and/or physical disease. *We will have unconsciously transformed energy into specific and unhealthy mass.*

A similar process occurs due to nontraumatic negative

events. If, for instance, a parent or teacher talks to us or treats us in some way that causes us to contract only slightly—a mildly negative event—then a single such instance, or even several, may have no long-term effect. But should this behavior continue over a long period of time, especially during our formative years, our habitual and oft-repeated contraction will incrementally cause a deep and malignant "energy scar."

While traumatic and negatively experienced events are unavoidable, their long-term destructive effects are not. In a healthy family or culture, the person who has undergone such a trauma may be immediately embraced and nurtured with compassion. There may be an outpouring of love and understanding. There may be physical treatments to encourage relaxation and the release of contracted energy. There may be meaningful dialogue, leading to important shifts in a relationship and/or actions to redress any wrongs and make corrections for the future.

Having passed through such a trauma and such subsequent healing, the individual will release the contracted energy, thus feeling immediately better, while circumventing any long-term problems. Furthermore, the event will have opened the person to a host of expanded, positive possibilities—he or she may well be stronger, wiser, healthier, or more loving. Indeed, the very intensity of the negative experience, with its great charge of excited energy, will determine just how positive the outcome can be.

When you are breathing, feel it, bodily and with emotion. Whatever you are *doing*, feel it altogether. Feel into all relations constantly.

If you are angry and too full of self-expression, inhale and receive and be vulnerable through all relations. . . . Then breathe evenly in the Happiness.

If you are sorrowful and full of self-pity, exhale, blow out the lungs, and bring energy, love, and strength into all your relations. . . . Then breathe evenly in the Happiness.

If you are afraid and full of doubt, breathe deeply and fully, with feeling. Breathe equally in and out, fully and clearly. Then breathe evenly in the Happiness.

Da Free John[7]

Every feeling is a field of energy. A pleasant feeling is an energy which can nourish. Irritation is a feeling which can destroy. Under the light of awareness, the energy of irritation can be transformed into an energy which nourishes.

Thich Nhat Hanh[8]

Breathe in deeply through the nose,
  filling your torso,
    and now breathe out through the mouth
    in a long, soft, gentle sigh.
Again, breathe in deeply through the nose,
  filling your torso with energy,
    and breathe out through the mouth
    in a long, soft, gentle sigh.
This time, breathe in through the nose,
  filling your torso, and now
    let the air out through the mouth, with a
    long sustained sound of aaaaaahhhhhh . . .
Again, breathe in through the nose,
  filling your torso, and
    breathe out through the mouth, with a
    long sustained sound of aaaaaahhhhhh . . .
Pause for a few moments,
  noticing any feelings or sensations.
Now continue for a minute or so,
  breathing in through the nose,
    filling yourself with energy,
    and letting the air go
    in a long, gentle aaaaaahhhhhh . . .
  as your eyes softly close . . .

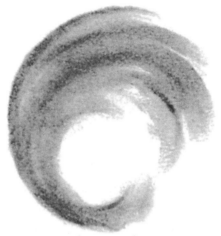

✳ IV ✳

The Dynamics of Response

Feelings are comprised of energy, and our capacity for feeling is a function of energy flow. Our greatest source of energy is breath, and our energy flow is determined mainly by the way in which we are breathing in any given moment.

This interrelationship between breath, energy, and feelings is a primary element in our lives—is indeed fundamental to the way in which we experience ourselves and to our powers of creation. The key to unleashing the full creative force of our feelings is in learning to consciously support through breathing the free, expansive flow of energy. Unfortunately, we typically learn to do precisely the opposite.

Remember how you breathe when you are very sad but trying hard not to cry. You will constrict your breathing, making it very shallow and preventing movement in your upper chest especially. You will also attempt to hold your lips tightly together, cutting off the flow of air along with any expression of sadness, though others may be able to detect a quivering in your chin.

Now remember how you breathe when you are trying hard not to get angry at someone you love. Again, a tightly controlled and contracted breath, usually along with a knot of tension in the solar plexus, tight bands of contracted muscle along the shoulders and neck, a clenched jaw, and a stiffened brow. Tense yourself in this way when you are feeling good, and then try to breathe. You cannot even approximate a good, free flow of breath once you have become so contracted.

Now remember how you breathe when you are trying hard not to laugh at an inappropriate moment. Yet more tightened muscles and stifled breath. And remember sitting through a tension-packed horror film. Or anticipating bad news at the doctor's office. Or sitting in a dentist's chair. Or late, and stuck in rush-hour traffic. Or watching the final moments of a nail-biting sporting event. Or attempting to suppress sexual excitement.

Once we begin to pay attention to our breath, and especially during moments of strong emotion, we notice that we are stopping and contracting the free flow of breath *all the time*—that, in fact, the most basic and automatic of human reactions to aroused feelings is to tighten the body and constrict the breath.

We do it because it is an effective short-term strategy for dealing with unwanted feelings. Feelings are comprised of energy, and energy flows through breath. If we are in the midst of feelings we do not want to experience, we can stop feeling by stopping the movement of energy—by stopping the breath.

Anytime we constrict our breath even slightly, we are diminishing the movement of energy throughout all levels of self. When we "turn down" the volume of energy, we are also turning off our awareness of feeling.

Let's return to the traumatic event. Faced with an urgently unwanted experience, we contract on all levels away from the event. We constrict our breathing and withdraw energetically, literally making ourselves as small as possible and reducing our vulnerability. We also reduce our present-time ability to feel the pain of the moment. This natural psychophysical reaction thus both protects us, somewhat, from further harm, while also relieving us, somewhat, from painful feelings.

Temporarily stopping such painful feelings, however, is not at all the same as healing the injuries that caused them. If we suppress our breathing until the event has ended, the pain has subsided, and we have gratefully begun to forget the injury, then we have only *suppressed* the pain—*we have not resolved it.* We are in fact carrying it within as a contracted energy scar—an "energy becoming mass" wound in our emotional body. If we are not taught to resolve such contractions—to breathe deeply, allowing our energies to expand, while consciously *feeling* the injury and opening to the necessary healing—then we shall carry the contraction as a part of who we are, quite possibly forever.

These contracted energy patterns affect us on all levels. They can manifest as mental neurosis or physical disease. They become interfering influences in all of our relationships. They define our perception of the world and greatly limit our possibilities.

Furthermore, they forever retain, as contracted energy, the

original unresolved feelings. Since breathing deeply and fully will always put us in touch with such unresolved feelings, we instinctively develop shallow, contracted breathing as a continuing condition in our lives. We learn to stay away—as breath, as energy—from these old hurts. When a present-time event in any way reminds us of an earlier, unresolved hurt, we immediately and habitually contract, breathing less, thus adding injury to injury.

Since breath is life, this short-term solution to unwanted feelings is slow suicide—an unconscious, moment-to-moment choice to feel less and to be less than fully alive.

As you grew up, people and events taught you to restrict the movement of your energy, the life within you. You are [now] hedged in by energetic habits that you know nothing about and that decide what you think life is like. They limit how much life you can know, how much pleasure you can feel, how passionately you can respond.

You can learn to have choices about what you're doing with your energy. This includes becoming aware of what your energetic habits are and developing the "energetic muscles" to free yourself from those habits. Voluntary energy distribution is a lot easier than you might think.

Julie Henderson[9]

There was a child went forth every day,
And the first object he look'd upon,
    that object he became,
And that object became part of him for the day
    or a certain part of the day,
Or for many years or stretching cycles
    of years.

Walt Whitman[10]

Breathing in and out through your nose,
let your inhale come softly and gently,
  filling your torso,
    and at the top of the inhale,
    without holding or stopping,
    release gently into the exhale, without
    effort or pushing, the air streaming out,
    and at the bottom of the exhale,
without any pause, breathe in again,
softly and gently, filling your torso,
  and at the top of the inhale,
    without holding or stopping,
    release gently into the exhale,
    the air softly streaming out,
    and at the bottom of the exhale,
    without any pause, breathe in again,
    softly and gently, filling your torso,
  and at the top of the inhale,
without holding or stopping,
 release gently into the exhale,
   the air softly streaming out,
    and without any pause, breathe in again,
    continuing for a few minutes,
    inhaling and exhaling, softly and gently,
    without stopping or pausing,
    as your eyes softly close . . .

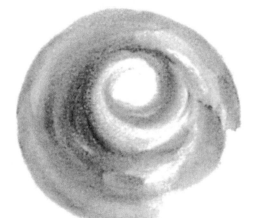

✳ V ✳

The Formation
of Primary Patterns

We learn to breathe at birth.
Those who are present—doctors, nurses, parents, and friends—
teach us how to breathe, though they rarely understand that they
are doing so. Because birth is such a powerfully challenging event,
bursting with emotional energy, the quality of our breathing lessons are critically important: we have passed through our first experience of stress, we have survived it, and within the first hour of
life we have established a fundamental relationship among energy,
breath, and feeling.

Under the very best of circumstances, birth is an intensely traumatic event. We have spent nine months in a warm and watery
heaven, only to be quite suddenly thrust into an alien world. The
womb that so wonderfully held and nurtured us becomes our
attacker. We are forced into a long, arduous, and terrifying labor—an absolute struggle for survival. Our bodies undergo extra-

ordinary pain from wave after wave of crushing contraction. For our psyches, there is equally extraordinary pain: we are being violently separated from all we have known, cut off from the source, and, truly, driven from the garden.

There is little in our adult lives that can even remotely compare to this primal ordeal (*giving* birth probably comes closest—or going off to war). For most of us, it is the nearest we will ever come to dying until the actual moment of our death. Furthermore, it may be the greatest test of our lives—the most challenging set of circumstances we will ever encounter—and the answers we find during such a test will naturally serve as our answers in all future tests; the lessons acquired at birth will become the foundations of our lifestyles and philosophies.

Though as infants we are obviously preverbal and physically undeveloped, we are nonetheless beings of great mental and emotional faculties. We see, hear, touch, taste, and smell; we form beliefs about the world based on our experiences; we develop attitudes and preferences; we learn to trust and not trust, to fear and not fear, to love and not love. We are thoroughly aware of the world around us, we are positively and negatively affected by the unique qualities of our world, and we grow as unique human beings according to the nature of our experiences.

Western science gives a totally different understanding of birth. It is thought that the fetus/newborn is somehow *pre*conscious and therefore unaffected, in any lasting way, by the circumstances of birth. Because an infant's brain is not yet fully developed, many scientists have reasoned that the human faculties of consciousness, emotion, memory, understanding, and learning are likewise undeveloped. In an astonishingly profound misunderstanding, they have looked at the newborn and concluded that *there is no one* there! There is a body, but not a person; pain, but not emotion; experience, but not memory; and awareness, but not learning.

Tragically, it follows that it does not really matter how you treat such a creature, so long as you are tending to her (or his) bodily survival. Since she is not yet a fully conscious being, she will not take offense or draw any conclusions from your behavior.

However, a body of research is beginning to substantiate what any mother already *knows*: that the newborn is conscious, intelligent, responsive, *and* impressionable.[11] Indeed, if anything, the newborn is *hyper*conscious—she has greater conscious awareness of the world in the first few hours of life than she shall likely have at any later time. While she will gradually develop unconscious mechanisms for screening out the vast quantities of sensory input to which she is forever exposed—she must do this to survive, to avoid sensory overload—as a baby she is wide open, totally receptive, and taking the whole world in through all of her senses.

Consequently, the newborn *will* suffer, as surely and meaningfully as any adult will suffer; she will respond to her suffering, like any adult, with the best of her capabilities; and she will learn and grow from such painful (and pleasurable) events—her present responses will be influenced by past experiences and will go on to influence future behavior.

Since the world is anything but perfect, the newborn will obviously experience some bad, unpleasant, and thoroughly unwanted events. However, she has a limited range of responses to such events: she cannot run, fight, verbally reason or intelligibly complain, or move to effectively alter a situation. Faced with a painful event, and unable to take effective action, she does the only thing she is able to: she constricts her breathing and contracts, *as energy*, away from the source of the pain. She pulls herself in—physically, mentally, emotionally, and energetically—disconnecting from the cause of her suffering and powerfully withdrawing from the hurtful world.

For just a moment, picture an emotionally suffering infant. Her contraction, on all levels, is obvious and easily felt. Though she may burst into crying—as a way of breathing fully, releasing the painfully pent-up energy, and demanding adult attention and assistance—she contracts away from the pain *first.* And while crying will often fully resolve the suffering—the energy is released and the situation is fixed by an adult—on too many occasions crying will not work and, indeed, will only make things worse, intensifying the pain and contraction.

It is important to understand that, *for the infant,* contraction of breath/energy in the presence of pain is a healthy, innate, and intelligent response. It is right and proper and critical to the infant's survival. It makes sense. And, if she is blessed with grown-ups who understand the dynamics of energetic response and know ways to encourage the relaxation and resolution of contracted energies, she will pass through her suffering well, while learning/growing in a healthy way into the future.

When she fails to receive such nurturing, however, and the hurt is extremely traumatic and/or often repeated, she will retain the contracted energy as a part of her experience. This fixed contraction of energy will affect her on all levels—as physical tension, as mental neurosis, and as emotional dysfunction. It will become a vital piece of the definition of her personality. And it will be a primary pattern through which she experiences the world and organizes her responses to future events.

For the baby, [the manner of birth] makes an enormous difference.

Whether we cut the umbilical cord immediately or not changes everything about the way respiration comes to the baby, even conditions the baby's taste for life.

If the cord is severed as soon as the baby is born, this brutally deprives the brain of oxygen.

The alarm system thus alerted, the baby's entire organism reacts. Respiration is thrown into gear as a response to aggression.

Entering life, what the baby meets is death. And to escape this death it hurls itself into respiration. The act of breathing, for a newborn baby, is a desperate last resort. Already the first conditioned reflex has been implanted, a reflex in which breathing and anguish will be associated forever. What a welcome into this world!

Dr. Frederick Leboyer[12]

Let your jaw hang open,
  and even as you read,
    breathe in and out through the mouth,
    with a light, gentle panting,
  a contented dog's breath,
letting all parts of the body remain
loose and relaxed, no effort to breathe,
  a light, gentle panting, the tongue loose
  and relaxed on the floor of the mouth,
    a light, gentle panting,
    a contented dog's breath,
feeling any sensations of body and mind,
a light, gentle panting, easy and rapid,
and continuing for a few minutes,
    feel any sensations,
      this light, gentle panting,
    this contented dog's breath,
as your eyes softly close . . .

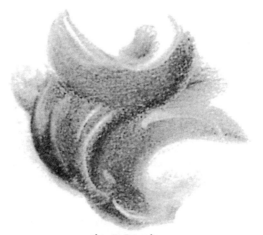

✳ VI ✳
Pain, Separation & the Habits of a Lifetime

Under the very best of conditions birth will involve a fair measure of suffering, which will in turn contribute to the psychophysical development of the new person. It is the responsibility of the attending adults to ease the way for the birthing infant as much as possible, and then to provide an environment that emanates warmth, safety, support, nurturance, and love. Ideally, the newborn's early lessons will be of monumental challenges well met, of painful contraction giving way to ecstatic release, and of the absolute presence of "motherlove"—the baby's experience of unconditional human and environmental support.

Such ideal conditions are rarely the case, however, and we all carry the unresolved pains of birth forward as we grow. If our culture has failed to recognize the connection between birth and human development, it is likely that we shall be burdened with

53

some especially painful, and negatively impactful, primal memories. Twentieth-century Western obstetrics—"techno-birthing," as I call it—dictates a particularly traumatic birth experience, with its own load of unnecessary burdens. It is generally useful, though somewhat unpleasant, to examine this approach to birth, as it has contributed so greatly to life as we currently know it.

This is not meant to question the integrity or the good intentions of those who practice Western obstetrics. They have been quite successful in sparing the mother pain and in keeping both the mother and infant physically alive. All of the procedures of techno-birthing have originated as legitimate reactions to life-threatening dangers that *sometimes* occur during birth. The problem is not that the technology of Western obstetrics is necessarily bad—much of it can and should be retained. Rather, it is that in failing to recognize the psychospiritual dimensions of life, birth has been made excessively traumatic, with dire developmental consequences for the infant.

The underlying assumptions of techno-birthing are that the natural process of childbirth cannot be trusted and that it is essentially and inherently dangerous. It is thought that from early in the pregnancy and on through the delivery both mother and infant are at considerable risk (not to mention the very real liabilities of the doctor). Birth is viewed as a medical emergency that calls for man-made interventions every step of the way.

It is significant to note that this viewpoint, and all of the interventions and procedures it has produced, are almost entirely the work of men, rather than women. For most of the world's cultures, and for most of Western history, birth has belonged quite rightly in the hands of women. The common sense of such an approach is clear: if we believe in birth as a natural, organic process, and if we trust that the woman's body that knows so well how to conceive and carry a child will also know how to deliver it, then it follows that other women will make the best midwives and that mothers will make the best of all.

Nevertheless, four hundred years ago, for reasons rooted in politics, religion, and economics, the Western world made a violent swing to absolute patriarchy. *Millions* of women throughout Europe and the Americas were murdered for the supposed crimes of witchcraft and heresy.[13] By the time this collective insanity had passed, the subjugation of an entire sex had been completed. There were no more women priestesses, teachers, or doctors—no more women in any positions of importance outside of the home (except for those women who practiced their craft in secrecy—hence the origin of the witch's coven). Perhaps most serious of all was the virtual disappearance of women midwives.

Let's examine such a situation. Take a culture that is already disinclined toward a fully sexual and ecstatic experience of the body. Add in a brutal prejudice against all things having to do with women. Allow it to stew for a couple of hundred years in a dominant theme of man versus nature, of "better living through modern chemistry," and top it off with the mistaken notion that infants are preconscious and unimpressionable. Then walk into a typical hospital delivery room and look at the results.

The interventions of techno-birthing often begin at the beginning: rather than wait for the infant/mother to initiate labor, contractions may be induced through chemical means.

Many babies are delivered according to doctor and hospital schedules, as if the organic timing of the mother/fetus/body has no relevance. The fetus is continuously monitored, in ways that often interfere with the mother's labor, and should the fetus's vital signs in any way fall outside of statistical norms, it is assumed that things are going wrong, and further interventions are undertaken. Unfortunately, each intervention tends to subvert the natural process, directly causing the need for further interventions.

The use of forceps, cesarean section, and/or anesthetics are all fairly standard procedures of techno-birthing to help the woman deliver, and each has its own often serious lasting effects for the infant. However he (or she) makes it out the womb, he is generally delivered into a world of chaotic sensory assaults: bright lights, loud voices, cold temperatures, harsh surfaces, masked faces—the perfect environment for surgery, perhaps, but a foolishly inhuman greeting for one who has spent nine months in the womb.

There are other horrors that may be visited upon this tiny new person, mostly in the name of sanitation and efficiency, such as the immediate separation of the newborn from his mother. (*How can we do this?*) But the greatest folly of all, and the one which causes the most long-term damage, is the premature cutting of the umbilical cord.

A lifetime of continuous breathing all begins with, and is conditioned by, the first breath out of the womb. It is a critical first step toward independence: to be able to breathe separately from the mother (she who has always breathed for the fetus, via the umbilical cord) is to establish oneself, in the most fundamental of terms, as an autonomous being. Breathing for oneself is the first step toward truly living free.

In addition, it is of the greatest importance that the newborn's brain receive a steady supply of oxygen. The transition from breathing with the umbilical cord to breathing with the lungs must be as smooth and uninterrupted as possible. Any oxygen deprivation during birth can have serious repercussions for the individual.

Nature, as we might have known, has provided more than adequate protection during this pivotal transition. The umbilical cord will continue to pulse with oxygen throughout the labor and for several minutes after the infant is born. It will continue to function, in fact, until the newborn has had the time to discover and slowly, slowly, establish full breathing with the lungs. When the umbilical cord is no longer needed, it will naturally stop functioning: the child will, in effect, cut his own cord. *He* will separate from his mother when *he* is ready.

All that is required for this first breath to spontaneously occur is patience and trust. When the process is unnecessarily aborted, an extreme emergency can result for the infant. Suddenly, oxygen is cut off—life is acutely threatened—and the infant has no innate capacity for responding to this event. He is moments from death and totally helpless. He explodes with panic!

Birth, at this point, is indeed a serious medical emergency, calling for radical emergency procedures. *The infant is grabbed by the heels, swung upside down, and struck—hard.* We can only shake our heads and wonder. Birth has been turned into a brutal and irrational torture and an initiation into violence. Learning to breathe has become the most traumatizing event of a person's life.

All of the terror of the moment is contained within that first breath. All of the infant's intensely contracted energy is contained within that first breath. All of his profound emotional pain is contained within that first breath. All of his screaming "I hate this!" is contained within that first breath.

The newborn is so powerfully influenced with this experience that a lifetime of shallow breathing may likely follow. A deep cellular connection between stress and breath has been impressed. And a host of painful and unresolved memories has been locked into the newborn's body as contracted breath/energy—the relevant data for the decisions, attitudes, patterns, and beliefs out of which he will create his life.

Imagine for a moment that you have just stepped off an airplane into some new and exotic country. The natives assault you with glaring light and deafening noise, and then they roughly manhandle and abuse your body. They seem calm, happy, perhaps even celebratory as they do all this. It would be the height of rationality to get back on the plane and fly away, firmly resolved to have nothing to do with such inhuman people.

Though we all chose to remain in *this* new and exotic place, can we really be blamed for many of our negative patterns and tendencies? If our natural intuitive responses are subverted from the very beginning, doesn't it make sense to grow distrustful of ourselves and irresponsible in our behavior? If the environment attacks us from the very beginning, doesn't it make sense to view the world as a hostile and unfeeling place? If the first person we ever meet inflicts violence upon us, doesn't it make sense to fear humanity and carry deep feelings of unsafety forward into future relationships? And if learning to breathe is a terrifying and panic-stricken event, then doesn't it make sense that we will instinctively avoid fully breathing for the rest of our lives?

The moment you breathe deeply, more energy becomes available in your body. Where there is energy flow, there is motion. You can experience this motion in many different ways: as sensations like tingling, numbness, or vibration, or as emotions such as sadness, joy, or anger, and finally as actual body movements that go with these emotions, like crying, laughing, or striking out. So, therefore, if you are afraid to feel, one of the most effective ways to keep yourself from feeling is to control your breathing.

Dr. Bruno Hans Geba[14]

By stimulating and directing positive, joyous feelings we can change the essence of our inner patterns and experience. When positive or joyous feelings and attitudes pass through each organ and circulate throughout our whole system, our physical and chemical energies are transformed and balanced. In other words, *we have the opportunity to recreate our bodies through positive energy.*

Tarthang Tulku[15]

Breathing in and out through the nose,
  feel your belly rising and falling
    with each breath, and, even as you read,
    continue to breathe deeply and slowly,
    while placing your awareness in the
  gentle rising and falling of the belly.
Notice that you can continue
  to read these words, while breathing gently
    in and out through the nose,
    and while feeling and enjoying
      the easy rising and falling of the belly,
      and continuing for a few minutes,
      feel and enjoy the coming and going of
      breath in your belly, rising and falling,
  as your eyes softly close . . .

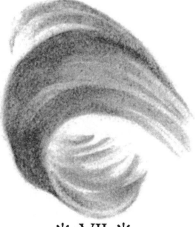

✳ VII ✳

Lessons in Breath

We learn to breathe at birth, even as we are learning about stress, emotion, and human relationship; even as we are exploring the nature of light, sound, touch, taste, and smell; and even as we are discovering the limits and possibilities of the human form. Birth is the beginning of all of our lessons, the first word in all of our intellectual development, and the genesis of our personal history.

This does not mean that we are rigidly determined by the circumstances of birth. There will be a continuing chain of new experiences, of traumatic, and joyous, events—a lifetime of new lessons, new growth, and new development. Still, to some degree, different with each person, everything that follows will be influenced and conditioned by the lessons of birth.

So much depends on the entirely unique environment into which each newborn lands. A terrifying birth followed by several days of uninterrupted motherlove—of mother holding, mother cooing, mother nursing, and mother caressing—will elicit very different lessons than a terrifying birth followed by several days of continuing rough treatment, abandonment, and pseudo food. (Could it be that the current prevalence of eating disorders is the instinctive response of the first generation to be routinely bottle-fed?) Infants who are greeted with violence and then surrendered to the warm, soft bodies of their mothers may learn that life here has its ups and downs, along with its good and not-so-good people. Infants who are greeted with violence and then left in a nursery with a bunch of screaming strangers may find themselves wondering, years later, why they feel so unsafe, so unwilling to trust, and so incapable of intimacy.

Any event that infants in any way dislike engenders the same fundamental response: energetic contraction away from the event. They do this initially to survive. With time and repetition, they learn that energetic contraction is also a successful strategy for eliminating unwanted feelings. They find that by contracting energetically—engineered primarily by suppressing breath—they can, in the present moment, lessen the intensity of unpleasant emotions.

As an example, infants who are struck will instinctively contract from the violating hand, will contract energetically from the unacceptable event, will contract emotionally from the awful feelings of shame, anger, and hate, and will contract their breathing as a way of retreating, becoming small, and hiding inside. They will do all of this immediately and automatically; they have no other means of response.

If this pain is not resolved, if these children are not encouraged and assisted in fully releasing from contraction, they will remain scarred by the event. Their nervous systems will be imprinted with the circumstances and with their reactions to those circumstances. They will carry the pain forward in the body as contracted energy, as emotional content, as conscious reflection, and as a specific manner of shallow breathing.

Though such violence is certainly extreme—and hopefully abnormal—infants' lives will always contain some negative events, no matter how conscientious their parents may be. The lessons of contraction are not aberrations; they are not caused by life gone wrong. Life will always provide unpleasant events, have moments of hurt, and contain the experience of pain. The challenge of birth, infancy, and early childhood is not that children be spared negative events, though we do the best we can; it is that they be *taught* to breathe and, thus, to fully resolve their pains, to release their contracted energies, to balance their emotions, and to consciously embrace life and all that it offers.

How can we teach breathing, if we ourselves have been mistaught? More to the point: if birth is indeed so very formative, then what can we—the aging misborn—do about it? Clearly, we cannot change the circumstances of our early years. If the tree must grow as the twig is bent, then what, if anything, can be done for the fully grown yet poorly bent tree?

The importance of examining the nature of birth is that we may better understand the source and dynamics of our patterned energy contractions. And in deeply understanding birth, it is also important that we, the parents and midwives of a coming generation, give our children a more humane and spiritually conscious beginning. It is not, however, necessary that we remember our own actual births or that we attempt to somehow deal with that experience as a *past* event.

Just as it is breath that specifically locks in the negative experiences of birth, so it is breath that can free us in this present moment. All of the contracted and unresolved patterns of our past are manifesting now, in present time, and they can be touched, felt, and transformed now, in present time, through simple conscious breathing. It is the continuing habit of shallow and contracted breathing that sustains our continuing habits of negatively contracted energy, and we can contact and encourage the release of any contracted energy through a single conscious moment of deep and flowing breath.

There are a great many approaches to conscious breathing, each of which will tend to have a specific technique and somewhat unique effect. However, most conscious breathing approaches are alike in that they stimulate an increase in quantity and flow/radiance of energy throughout the body and mind.

This increase in *moving* energy leads to a direct experience of any stuck and *unmoving* energy. The individual breather thus becomes immediately aware of how she or he is most critically blocking the free movement of energy. The person feels it now, in present time. Typically, the present-time awareness of such a block is unpleasant. It hurts—physically, emotionally, and/or mentally.

The free movement of energy, in contrast with the painful awareness of contracted energy, becomes a growing edge of transformation. The individual directly experiences habits of the past and the capacity for change in the present moment. In consciously breathing for the space of a minute or so, a person increases the free movement of living energy throughout the many levels of self, which allows him or her to tangibly *feel*, in present time, specific patterns of contracted energy. While such patterns usually have their origins in early events, and while awareness of such patterns will often trigger vivid memories, the breather's immediate experience of contracted energy—how does it feel, *right now*—carries, and turns, the key to positive transformation.

Breath—breathing, breathing, breathing—*is* the key.

It has been known for centuries that it is possible to induce profound changes of consciousness by techniques which involve breathing. The procedures that have been used for this purpose by ancient and non-Western cultures cover a very wide range from drastic interferences with breathing to subtle and sophisticated exercises of the various spiritual traditions. Thus the original form of baptism as it was practiced by the Essenes involved forced submersion of the initiate under water, which typically brought the individual close to death by suffocation. This drastic procedure induced a convincing experience of death and rebirth, a far cry from its modern form involving sprinkling of water and a verbal formula. In some other groups, the neophytes were half-choked by smoke, by strangulation, or by compression of the carotid arteries. Profound changes in consciousness can be induced by both extremes in the breathing rate—hyperventilation and prolonged withholding of breath—or a combination of both.

Stanislav Grof [16]

Breathe in and out through the nose, and,
even as you read, feel or sense or imagine
that with every inhale you can draw energy
in through the entire surface of your body.
Simply imagine that each slow, deep,
inhaled breath is drawing energy in
through every cell of your body,
that the whole outer surface of your skin
opens to and receives energy
with each deep inhaled breath.
And, even as you read,
feel or sense or imagine
that with every exhale
you are radiating energy outward,
like a glowing light or a burning flame,
with every exhale the entire surface of
your body releases energy, radiates energy.
Continue breathing in through the skin,
and radiating out through the skin,
breathing in through the skin,
and radiating out through the skin,
for a few minutes more,
as your eyes softly close . . .

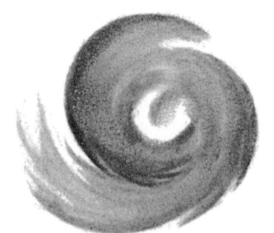

✳ VIII ✳

The Circle of Breath

The simplest and most direct way to experience the full promise and power of the breath is through a pattern that is often called "circular breathing." In circular breathing, one breathes in a continuous flow, without interruption or pause, for an extended period of time. The inhale leads directly to the exhale, without the breather stopping or holding the breath in; and the exhale leads directly to another inhale, without any pause between breaths. The inhale and the exhale are connected, flowing easily from one into the other, allowing for one continuous flow of breath—inhaling into exhaling into inhaling—and thus creating the image of a moving circle of breath/energy.

With just a few minutes, more or less, of circular breathing, any of a wide range of effects may begin to occur. The breather may feel a warm tingling sensation in the hands, face, or feet, which may spread quite wonderfully throughout the body. Or the tingling may intensify, typically, into a tight and extremely painful cramping of muscles, first in the hands, then face, then feet, then elsewhere.

The breather may become faint or light-headed and have difficulty remaining focused. There may be long periods of time in which one barely breathes at all and in which all breathing seems a great effort.

The breather may experience nausea, choking, muscle tremors, or sudden extremes of hot and/or cold temperatures. Any part or system of the body that has ever been injured, damaged, or felt as inadequate is likely to become hypersensitive through continuous circular breathing.

The breather may remember his or her birth with extraordinary clarity or may remember any number of early experiences, including prenatal life in the womb. These memories may come as visual images, or they may be apparent in the actual movements and expressions of the breather's present-time body.

The breather will undoubtedly *feel* with great intensity. Sadness, shame, rage, fear, feelings of being out of control, feelings of vulnerability, feelings of helplessness, feelings of stark terror—such emotions can rush like waves through the breather, threatening to swallow up and overwhelm. Indeed, one of the more useful images during circular breathing is that of *riding the rapids*, the rapids being the emotional intensity that continuous circular breathing invariably releases.

More encouragingly, the breather may experience body tingling that excites into ecstatic joy; waves of sexual pleasure surging *everywhere*; a profoundly deep relaxation; powerful insights into the nature of life; visions of deep, mystical content; or an unforgettable spiritual rebirth. And the breather may discover, *at the cellular level*, the essential connection between breath, emotion, and energy.

Western medical scientists have observed these effects (the less pleasant effects especially) and lumped them all under the rubric of "hyperventilation syndrome," explaining that when one breathes too rapidly or continuously it upsets the normal exchange of oxygen and carbon dioxide, which in turn causes these negative difficulties. The standard "cure" is to cut down on the sufferer's oxygen intake (often by placing a bag over the head) until the condition has subsided. The implication, of course, is that breathing too much is unhealthy, if not dangerous.

The fact that hyperventilation syndrome most often occurs spontaneously to those under great stress has gone unexplained by such scientists. Likewise, the positive benefits of hyperventilation have been ignored completely, as have the reports from long-time practitioners of circular breathing that indicate that if one sustains deep, continuous breathing for long enough the negatively contracting experiences will give way to expansive joy.

Hyperventilation is not a negative syndrome, but a positive solution: it is the cure to a lifetime of subventilation. When practiced intentionally, hyperventilation floods the body/mind with great rushes of energy, causing a powerful release and cleansing of contracted energies.[17]

For others (often children) who may never have thought of breath or energy, the compounding stresses of daily living may one day push them too painfully into excessive contraction and *the body will attempt to heal itself* by breathing deeper and faster—it will hyperventilate. The tragedy is not that such people are subjected to a bothersome syndrome; the tragedy is that their experiences are misunderstood and their potential healings are stifled, mislabeled, and turned into cause for further contraction.

Western medicine will fail to understand breath and the effects of deep breathing so long as it fails to understand the movement of energy within the human experience. Indeed, trying to understand breath without an awareness of energy is like trying to understand the heart without an awareness of blood. Hyperventilation, in all its forms and effects, can be understood only within the context of moving and contracted energy/emotion.

Circular breathing works by creating a strong, flowing circuit of energy throughout the body and mind. As energy flows with greater and greater intensity, the breather becomes aware of specific patterns of contracted, unflowing energy. Because such patterns of contraction are rooted in painful experiences, the present-time awareness typically hurts, at first.

Any of the "negative" effects described above may occur—and usually with great intensity due to the great charges of energy involved. The simple and well-demonstrated power of circular breathing is this: If the breather keeps breathing, the continuing flows of energy will wash through and open the patterns of contraction, bringing lightness where there was density, softening and relaxing the hard, painful places in the person's experience, and turning old emotional hurt into radiant, loving joy.

We have been able to confirm repeatedly Wilhelm Reich's observation that psychological resistances and[1] defenses use the mechanisms of restricting the breathing. Respiration has a special position among the physiological functions of the body. It is an autonomous function, but it can also be easily influenced by volition. Increase of the rate and of the depth of breathing typically loosens the psychological defenses and leads to release and emergence of the unconscious (and superconscious) material.

Stanislav Grof[18]

[Rebirthing, or circular breathing] is not teaching a person how to breathe, it is the intuitive and gentle act of learning how to breathe from the breath itself. It is connecting the inhale with the exhale in a relaxed intuitive rhythm until the inner breath, which is the Spirit and source of breath itself, is merged with air—the outer breath.

Leonard Orr[19]

Breathe in and out through the nose,
  allowing your breath to come and go
  in an easy four-beat rhythm,
breathe in through the nose, three, four
  now hold the breath in, three, four
    breathe out through the nose, three, four
    now pause between breaths, three, four
breathe in through the nose, three, four
  now hold the breath in, three, four
    breathe out through the nose, three, four
    now pause between breaths, three, four
breathe in through the nose, three, four
  now hold the breath in, three, four
    breathe out through the nose, three, four
    now pause between breaths, three, four
continue to breathe, in this easy rhythm,
  for several more minutes, three, four
  as your eyes softly close . . .

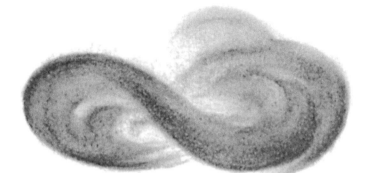

❊ IX ❊

Partners in Breath

While deep, circular breathing is the simplest of techniques, the process it enables is not always easy. Resolving the strong patterns of contraction that we invariably embody and sustain as a condition of living can be difficult and at times overwhelming.

As a rule, we will bring to awareness only those issues and energies we are capable of successfully resolving in the present moment. This is a safety clause for the individual breather: you cannot hurt yourself breathing,[20] but you may be able to go only so far alone.

For our deepest work it seems important, and perhaps necessary, to breathe with a partner or guide. It may be that since our patterns of contraction are rooted in relationships with other humans, we need the presence of a human relationship to generate and *feel together* transformation and wholeness. It certainly is true that having a hand to hold, a shoulder to cry on, and a calm reassuring voice can make a powerful difference.

There are a number of groups and individuals working with circular breathing, or close variations, and a beginning breather would do well to connect with an experienced guide, if possible. It also can be quite empowering for two sincere and like-minded individuals to be guides, one to the other, through the aches and joys of circular breathing. What follows are practiced rules of thumb that can govern and support the process of those who choose to work together.

The setting for breathing sessions is very important. Ideally, it should be as womblike as possible; thus, indoor settings tend to work better than outdoor settings, and small rooms tend to work better than larger rooms. The space should be quiet, private, warm, and entirely safe, both physically and psychologically. There must be no question of interruptions: no telephones ringing, no pets barking, no roommates wandering through, no children needing attention. There should be water, tissues, and blankets readily at hand. Finally, both partners should be wearing loose, comfortable clothing that easily allows deep breathing, and belts, jewelry, eyeglasses, and watches should be removed.

The breathing partner, or breather, should recline with eyes closed for the duration of the session. It is best to breathe in and out through the mouth, as this enables the greatest flow of breath/energy. There is, however, no need for strenuous exertion; rather, it is enough to breathe just a little bit deeper and little bit faster than usual, while settling into a steady, sustained rhythm. Breathing in and out through the mouth, making just enough effort to increase one's energy experience, and sustaining a rythmic effort for an extended period (fifteen to sixty minutes) will initiate the changes appropriate at any given time. The breather is encouraged to lie as still as possible, allowing the body to sink into relaxation. Likewise, the breather is encouraged to "stay inside," verbally quiet, paying close attention to physical sensations and the excitement of feelings.

During those times when "nothing seems to be happening," the breather needs to continue breathing, while attending closely to sensations and feelings. Likewise, during those times of intense physical and/or emotional experience, the breather needs to continue breathing, as the breath provides the steady support needed to move through and resolve such experiences.

Finally, the breather is encouraged to release the exhale, neither restricting its movement (letting it out in a narrow stream) nor forcefully blowing it out. The body is designed to exhale by itself, requiring no added effort. If the breather will give effort only to the inhale, pulling the air in, and then release all effort (surrender), a full exhale will naturally follow, leading in turn to the next inhale.

Throughout the process, the most basic instruction for the breather remains: breathe and feel, breathe and feel. To which must be added: trust the process.

Within minutes, any of a wide spectrum of experiences may come to awareness, such as physical sensations, vivid memories, random thoughts, visual images, or strong emotions. The challenge for the breather is always the same: stay with the breath; accept everything as the free movement of energy; stay with the breath.

Simple though it may sound, there are times when continuing to breathe can be quite difficult. It is for such moments that a partner, or sitter, is needed.

The sitter's role is precisely that: to sit, to be totally there for the breather, and to be an active witness in another's growth. In many sessions, that is all that will be needed. The time will pass in silence, as the breather moves through various changes toward ever-expanding clarity and joy. For such sessions it is enough that the sitter breathe with the breather, providing the most intimate and tangible kind of support: breathing as one with the other person.

In other sessions, the sitter may take a more active role.[21] The sitter should always be ready to provide water, tissues, and blankets as needed. If the breather begins moving around, the sitter may provide support, as well as protection, from falling off of a bed, for instance, or bumping into objects. In this regard, the sitter guarantees the continuing safety and support of the environment.

The sitter may be moved to touch the breather, in a variety of ways ranging from simple hugs to the laying on of hands. If the sitter is skilled in any bodywork or healing disciplines, then extended hands-on support may be appropriate. With or without such skill, any loving touch—from the heart and with a genuine desire to help—may certainly further the breather's progress.

There also are times when talking helps or, at least, when listening to the breather's experience helps. Any of a wide range of verbal therapies can prove useful during a breathing session, depending on the skills of the sitter.

The main problem with both touch and talk is that they may easily come to be relied on too much, becoming well-intended distractions from the breath. An important lesson of circular breathing is that we can heal ourselves through the primary and immediately accessible activity of breath. To add too much "non-breath" to a session might leave one with the sense that it was the bodywork or the special abilities of the sitter that caused the transformation.

Each new therapeutic input the sitter uses to help the breather tends to remove both breather and sitter from the simple power of the breath. Thus, the most basic instruction for the sitter is also to breathe and feel, while absolutely trusting the simplicity of the process.

A second problem with adding other modalities (touch, dialogue, music) to a breathing session is that the sitter may become too involved in trying to "fix" the breather. In a way not dissimilar to techno-birthing, each intervention from the sitter tends to subvert the breather's inherent healing potential, while making the sitter more and more responsible for the breather's process.

A good guideline, then, for the sitter is to allow only short stretches of touch or talk, always returning to the breath, encouraging the breather to "breathe it for a while now." The most constant contribution of the sitter should always be variations on the theme of "breathing and feeling, breathing and feeling."

The sitter has no easy task. To sit for long silent periods, offering nothing more than a loving breath, calls for great patience. And during those times when heavy contracted energies are emerging (emergencies), it often requires the most courageous leap of faith to trust that the breath can carry us through.

Fortunately it can, and it always will.

All these symptoms appear and disappear in a matter of minutes. All one has to do is maintain connected breathing. . . . These symptoms are caused by past thoughts and feelings. A symptom is the manifestation of an old negative thought in your body so that you can release it through your breath. *All symptoms are the cure in process.* A negative thought, formerly suppressed, is trying to get out. It is much better to go through a few minutes of symptoms and breathe it out than it is to have those negative thoughts suppressed and causing negative mental mass (disease). The symptoms are rarely very painful unless you start making them real. All they really are is thoughts that you can change. Most people, in fact, think of these dramatic psychophysical memory phenomena as interesting and even fun. The symptom is a real body sensation, but a continued breathing rhythm causes it to disappear in a few minutes. Your breath and spirit releases the symptom from your mind and body, and you feel free and clear.

Leonard Orr[22]

Begin by forcefully blowing the air
out of your lungs, and now STOP,
  no breathing in, simply holding the breath out,
  as relaxed as you can, paying attention to
  all feelings and sensations, acutely aware
  of a life without breath, for as long as
you can, until it's time to breath in . . .
And breathe normally now, in an out through
  the nose, paying attention to all feelings
  and sensations, even as you read, for a
  few long, slow breaths, paying attention
  to all feelings and sensations . . .
And blow the air forcefully out of your lungs
  and now STOP, no breathing in, simply holding
  the breath out, as relaxed as you can,
  while paying attention to all feelings
  and sensations,
  acutely aware of a life without breath,
  for as long as you can,
until it's time to breathe in . . .
And breathe normally now, for several
  slow breaths, and for the next few minutes
  simply pay attention to all
  feelings and sensations,
  as your eyes softly close . . .

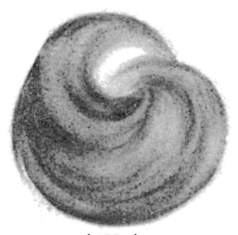

✳ X ✳

Rapture, Excitement & the Lessons of Sleep

Recall the dynamics of contracted energy. We are faced with a challenging experience that we cannot or will not accept; we generate energy to respond to the challenge, while simultaneously contracting through breath, as energy—from the event; and the immediate choice of contraction, unresolved, becomes a part of who we are: a physical, mental, and emotional pattern of held tension through which we experience the world and react to future events.

Circular breathing brings us into direct contact with our patterns of contraction while at the same time providing the means for their resolution. The process of resolution tends to move in one of three basic directions. The first, and most prevalent, is toward rapture. The breath initiates a gentle and thoroughly enjoyable release of long-held energies that is personal, self-informing, and deeply healing. The other two possibilities, which can be seen as paths, or preambles, to rapture, are *intensity* and *phasing out.*

During periods of *intensity,* the breather is contacting and exciting strong flows of contracted energy. There may be overwhelming—and quite dramatic—feelings of sadness, rage, shame, fear, or sexual arousal. There may be equally dramatic physical reactions: hot and cold flashes, nausea, choking, the uncontrollable shaking of body parts, and, quite often, extreme muscular cramping in the face, arms, hands, legs, and feet. Such emotional and/or physical intensity can be painful and, at times, rather frightening.

The common and instinctive tendency during intensity is to express oneself: through crying, moaning, or screaming; through physical movements such as shaking the head or pounding the fists; or by struggling against the body's reactions and efforting to make them stop. Such expressions generally are reflections of the emerging pattern of contraction; that is, the breather is reliving the very way in which full energetic resolution was originally avoided.

Rather than expressing during intense moments, the breather is encouraged to *keep breathing* and, thus, to truly feel what is happening. A basic discovery is that *expressing* one's emotions (or physical tensions) and *feeling* one's emotions/tensions are two entirely different activities. Indeed, we find that we simply cannot continue crying or screaming or physically struggling while at the same time sustaining a steady flow of breath.

Expression occurs in the extremities—the face, arms, and legs—and is a way of expending the excess charge of contracted energy. We feel purged after strenuous expression, which is certainly better than holding tension inside. But expression rarely gets to the root of a contracted pattern and thus is only a short-term fix.

As an analogy, when a teapot on a hot burner reaches the boiling point, it expresses its excess charge by blowing off steam. While this keeps the pot from exploding, it obviously does nothing to affect the source of the steam. So it is with the expression of energetic tension: it is better than exploding or increasing tension, but it is not the same as fully resolving the source pattern of contraction.

To fully resolve our patterns of contraction, we must sustain a flow of breath/energy while committing ourselves to absolute feeling in the present moment. While expression happens in the extremities, feeling happens in the torso and is continuously influenced by the breath. Through deep, conscious breathing the root of the energetic intensity—the pattern itself—is touched, moved, and finally resolved. Breathing keeps us right in the heart of energetic intensity until we contact the actual source of the contraction—a choice made in the past—and we can consciously choose to be different, by continuing to breathe, here and now, in the present moment. The power of this fresh choice is such that the most dramatic emotional and physical experiences can suddenly change to deep and peaceful relaxation—rapture—in the space of a few breaths.

When breathing alone, you will tend to go only so far into intensity. It is important to be gentle with yourself—and patient. If the experience becomes too intense to handle, slow the breath and, as soon as possible, stand up and move around.

Affirm that some work has been done and that eventually the time will be right to go further.

It is much easier to resolve intense patterns of contraction when breathing with a partner. The sitter can provide physical and emotional support, as well as constant encouragement to stay with the breath. It is rather logical for the breather, caught up in the throes of physical and emotional intensity, to think, "Breathing caused this, so I had better stop breathing!" The sitter is there to gently remind the breather to keep breathing: "You are doing great; your body is safe; *stay with the breath, open to your feelings.*"

The sitter can also guide the breather, when appropriate, to a specific pattern of circular breathing that can help during especially intense moments: a quick and shallow panting breath, focused in the center of the chest. This breathing pattern is similar to that which women learn for resolving pain during childbirth, and it is an excellent way to ride the waves of energetic intensity to full resolution.

Most importantly, the sitter must remain calm during periods of intensity. More precisely, the sitter must *exude* calm— he or she must communicate, on every level, reassurance, encouragement, and implicit trust in the process. However dramatic the breather's experience may be, the sitter cannot get caught up in reacting to an emergency. Rather, the sitter must compassionately, and with the gentlest of care, extend love to that which is emerging.

Phasing out occurs when the breather shifts to sub- or supraconscious levels of awareness: he or she phases out of conscious, present-time, embodied awareness to any of a number of alternate states. The breath becomes almost imperceptibly quiet, with long pauses between the exhale and the inhale. The body stills, as in deep sleep, though it may sporadically jerk and twitch, a condition called "myo-flexing."

During periods of phasing out, the breather is only vaguely aware of the breath. Likewise, the breather feels somewhat disembodied or feels at most a physical numbness or does not feel at all. There is a sense of drifting in and out of consciousness: the breather takes a dozen or so long, slow breaths and then slips away. After a time, the breather may come back into focus, pick up with the breathing again, and then, again, after a few breaths, phase out.

While there is little physical or emotional activity during periods of phasing out, there may be a wide array of internal experiences. The breather may pass through vivid dream sequences or memories, often relating to childhood and/or birth. There may be extraordinary spiritual experiences: of traveling out of the body, of meetings with angels or guides, of bright lights and wondrous colors, or of beautiful sounds. Or the breather may experience "nothing" at all—just having phased into deep and relaxing sleep.

In terms of contracted patterns of energy, phasing out indicates either a direct and gentle flow to rapture or a patterned avoidance of intensity. In the first case, the breather has contacted patterns of contraction and has easily moved to rapture. It is vital to understand that rapture is our birthright—our essential ground of being—and is, potentially, always just a breath away.

A common therapeutic trap is that of "no pain, no gain"—the idea that in order to grow one *must first* pass through hardship. This belief can be especially ingrained in one who has had a profound breakthrough experience that began with intense pain: a growth pattern can be established in which any easy and painless growth is distrusted or discounted. Though we must be prepared for and accepting of the pains and trials of intensity, we must also gratefully embrace joy in any moment it arises. And joy will often arise through the simple encouragement of several deep, conscious breaths.

On the other hand, phasing out is often an avoidance pattern: the breather has contacted a pattern of contraction and shifted to another level of awareness rather than experience the intensity—and challenges—of excited energy. Most everybody has some such avoidance patterns that will eventually come to awareness through conscious breathing. Those who were born under the effects of drugs, or had great difficulty breathing at birth (especially "blue babies," premature babies, and/or those who were placed in incubators), or have had a history of alcohol or drug abuse will face the greatest challenges with phasing out as avoidance.

Phasing out entails shifting away from conscious awareness, and as such it lowers one's capacity for conscious choice. Thus, when breathing alone, there is little one can do about phasing out other than allowing oneself to thoroughly enjoy the effects of deep peace, reverie, and relaxation. If every period of deep breathing leads to phasing out, then it is likely that one is avoiding and will need the support of a partner.

The sitter faces two choices when the breather is phasing out. The first is to sit quietly and allow the experience to unfold. This is generally a good idea if it is the first time the breather is phasing out, as it is beneficial to follow the breather's unique process. Also, a breather will often emerge suddenly from a sustained period of phasing out exploding with great intensity; the sitter must give this the space to happen—and in its own time. Finally, if there is a great deal of myo-flexing occurring—sporadic spasms indicating the spontaneous release of contracted energies—it is good to allow this for a while, as it has profound healing implications for the breather.

However, when phasing out recurs (indicating a reactive pattern) or when the body is totally still (indicating a dense unconsciousness, much like anesthesia), the sitter's role is to encourage the breather to stay in the body, to remain conscious, to keep breathing, and to feel.

The more caught up in an avoidance pattern the breather is, the more difficult it can be to return to conscious awareness and *to want to breathe*. The root of most avoidance patterns is abdication, quitting: "I don't want to." It is the easy surrendering of one's will during a negative event, rather than the intense activity of struggle.

The sitter is in effect providing a measure of will for the phasing-out breather. The gentle repetitions of "Keep breathing; stay in your body, open to your feelings" are often enough to keep the breather focused. Having the breather breathe with eyes open for a stretch and/or having the breather sit up works very well. Also, having the breather talk about his or her experience for awhile will refocus the process in present time, providing a "stepping off" place for further breathing.

The challenge with phasing out—as avoidance or rapture—is for the breather to become focused, alive, alert, and present, in the body now, and *within* the choice to breathe again, and again, and again.

Finally, it is important that any possible interventions be cleared with the breather in advance of the session so that they will be experienced, in present time, as functions of the breather's intention. Most of our patterns of contraction stem from *well-intentioned* subversions of the will by others at earlier times. Thus, the most well-intentioned interventions by the sitter—if not chosen by the breather—may only strengthen the breather's patterns of contraction.

Whether we are breathing alone or with a partner, whether exploding with intensity or phasing out, if there is any question of how to proceed we can always err well on the side of doing less: breathing again, open to feeling, and trusting the process as it uniquely unfolds.

Because both external and internal energies come from the same "breath" or "prana," as our inner environment changes, our relationship with the external world changes too, and the universe becomes much more comfortable to be in. It is as if the outer world of objects and our inner world of the senses—our consciousness—were to merge. We support the world, and it supports us and our senses. Our senses give us pleasure, and we feel positive; we project that, and receive back what we project. Inner and outer become harmonized and balanced.

Tarthang Tulku[23]

Before [world peace] happens there will be many tribulations, volcanic eruptions, the terrestrial atmosphere of our everyday life will change, what with poisonous vapors, virus chemicals, and at last—a Famine of Breath—

Only those who know *how to breathe* will survive.

Pundit Acharya[24]

Breathing in and out through your mouth,
with the jaw hanging loosely open, and
your breathing slow, quiet, calm, gentle,
even as you read feel your belly
moving with each breath,
expanding gently with each inhale,
drawing in life, and releasing gently
with each exhale, letting life go,
every inhale, filling your belly,
and every exhale, letting go . . .
Now allow yourself to breathe in and out
through your nose and mouth at the same
time so that exactly the same amount of air
is passing in and out through both openings,
while continuing to source each breath
from deep in your belly.
And for the next few minutes,
continue this breathing,
equal amounts of air passing
through your nose and mouth,
your belly gently rising and falling
with each easy breath,
as your eyes softly close . . .

The Continuing Process
of Resolution

The underlying question we have been addressing all along is "How do people change?"

If we assume the possibility of arriving in this life free, unencumbered, and divinely alive with joyous potential, then how do we become so stress ridden, so psychologically bound, and so physically and emotionally contracted? And if we acknowledge such patterns of contraction as unnecessary limitations, then *how do we change*? Is it possible to transform our habitual pains and weaknesses into present-time pleasures and strengths?

We have learned that through unconscious choices—enacted and embodied as unconscious breathing patterns—we have too often contracted from the fullness of life. Owing to prevailing environmental and human-relational constraints, we may have had no other options: we did the best we could with bad situations, quite rightly contracting ourselves as breath/

energy. We chose survival, in the only way possible to us at the time.

Every choice to contract, however unconscious or justly defensive, changes us—it is an act of self-change—and too often for the worse. Sadly, we mostly fail to resolve such choices, and, sadly, we carry our patterns of contraction forward into the present moment, while setting the stage for future unhappiness.

We are also learning that the breath that has bound us can set us free again: that the simple, sustained practice of conscious breathing can touch and move and finally resolve our long-held tensions, releasing strong currents of living energy and opening us to a world of vibrant, rapturous possibilities. Thus, our changes, for good and for ill, are functions of personal solutions to the events of our lives, which are in turn reflected in and affected by our moment-to-moment manner of breathing.

All of our patterns of contraction functioned in the moment of their conception as solutions to the dynamics of a specific event. Energetic contraction was a way of solving the inherent difficulties of the event and, aside from the future consequences, worked very well.

"Resolution" derives from the Latin *resolvere*, meaning "to solve anew." To resolve our patterns of contraction is to recognize that as solutions to life's problems such patterns are no longer viable, or wanted, and then to take steps to consciously "solve anew."

The dictionary gives two pertinent definitions of "resolution": (1) the process of resolving something or breaking it up into its constituent elements, and (2) a determined solving, as of a puzzle, or answering, as of a question; a solution.

The process of resolution—via sustained, conscious

breathing—generally passes through each of the above meanings: first there is an emergence of some of the constituent elements of a contracted pattern, and then there is the conscious and determined choice of a new solution.

In earlier chapters, we have examined the myriad of constituent elements that may come to the awareness of a conscious breather. The physical movements and reactions, the waves of emotion, the thoughts and insights, the internal visions, the memories, the sexual feelings—these are all pieces of the original "story" behind the pattern of contraction. The breather comes into contact with an old pattern, and specific elements of the pattern, relating to the source event in question, begin to emerge.

Thus, one who was delivered with forceps may experience a headache while feeling quite enraged. One who was abused as a child may feel sudden overwhelming shame, then rage, and may be alternately pleased and strongly displeased by any touching that a partner offers. One who started life in an incubator may need another blanket—and another, and another—feeling an intense need to be hot and enclosed. And one whose cord was cut prematurely may gasp for breath, as the throat tightens and fills with phlegm.

Old, forgotten injuries may come to sudden memory—may even hurt physically—while the event is recalled. Or conscious memory may be vague and insubstantial, while intense physical and emotional "memory" plays out: the breather who curls into a fetal position, feels totally panic stricken, and pushes urgently with the top of the head against a sitter's hand; or the breather who starts to feel sexually aroused, only to abruptly phase out into dense and unconscious sleep.

While we may question whether these constitute real memories of actual events, their absolute relevance to the breather are beyond doubt. As each piece emerges, the breather *knows* that it is real—and important. Furthermore, obvious correlations between past and present relationships, past and present events, and past and present personal tendencies come readily to awareness, and with all the power of incisive insight.

The purpose of the emerging memory, however, is not that the "whole story" be known or relived. The breather who insists on total recall of an event will likely be disappointed and will very likely frustrate the process of resolution. For reasons rooted in mystery, we are usually given specific pieces of our puzzle and nothing more. Fortunately, a single piece can suffice.

The purpose of an emerging memory, in whatever way it is experienced, is that it connects us to the feelings / energy / breath of the original event. We have breathed into contact with a pattern of contraction, the energy has moved, a piece of the pattern has emerged into present-time awareness, and we are now able to *feel again* a critical moment of past choice.

Once we are in touch with the feelings of the pattern, the story behind it becomes unimportant. Indeed, once the feelings are revived, the past itself is irrelevant. All that matters is occurring in present time, can be experienced in present time, and can be effectively resolved in present time.

The choice to contract is palpable, self-evident, and immediately relevant within the emerging feelings: "I can't breathe! I don't want to breathe! You can't make me breathe! I don't like this! I don't want this! Make it stop! I can't go on!" We are actually *living* a primal choice and its consequences, and the opportunity to resolve that choice—to solve it anew—is present. We can keep breathing, while allowing the feelings: we can consciously choose to stay open, inspired, and expanding. We can reach, through the past, for present joy and rapture.

This is the process of resolution: through sustained conscious breathing, we touch, move, and once again feel our old, destructive, and long-forgotten hurts. We feel the choices that changed us into contracted, limited beings, and we feel, breathe, and embody fresh choices: we choose to change in ways appropriate to our current lives, rather than living out of the scars and traumas of the past.

The uniquely human function of sexuality is not reproduction but ecstasy. It is the unification of the separate physical, emotional, and mental functions through a total release of reactivity—and it is the sacrifice of the whole and entire bodily and independent being through the awakening of total psychophysical feeling, or love.

Truly human lovers become a sacrifice to one another, and through one another to Infinity, in the very cycle of their breathing. All motion, all tension, all degenerative urgency, and all localization of feeling and attention in the genitals alone are mastered through awareness and feeling as the whole and entire bodily being. That free, unobstructed, nonreactive, and intense feeling is to be breathed to the entire bodily being in every cycle of breath, during sexual embrace and also in every moment of living.

Da Free John[25]

Breathing in and out deeply
  through your mouth,
    with the jaw hanging loosely open,
    and your breathing deep, slow, calm,
    and gentle, even as you read
     become aware of the perineum,
     a small area of skin and muscle located
     between the anus and the genitals,
   which is sometimes called the lunar point.
Continue to breathe deeply,
  in and out through the mouth,
    your belly gently rising and falling,
    simply paying attention to the lunar point,
     simply being aware of the place between
     your anus and genitals, and
      notice that it is easy to breathe deeply,
      easy as your belly rises and falls
     to also pay attention to the lunar point,
    to be gently focused and aware
  with each easy breath.
And for the next few minutes, continue this
  breathing deep and slow through the mouth,
    paying attention to the lunar point,
     focused at the lunar point,
     as your eyes gently close . . .

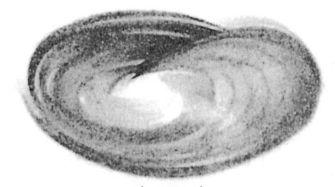

✳ XII ✳

Sexual Energy
& the Energetic Embrace

Deep, flowing breath is essentially arousing and exciting. Though we may breathe through periods of phasing out, such periods are always stages along the way to greater rapture. Recovering the full power and promise of the breath ultimately means generating and embodying strong flows of living energy, thus opening oneself to ever-expanding vibratory awareness and, finally, committing oneself to wondrously ecstatic sexual communion *as a fundamental condition of being alive.*

To the interconnected relationship of breath, energy, and emotion that we have already described, we must now add a fourth ingredient: the individual's awareness and experience of sexual energy. The way that an individual sexually develops is a primary pattern affecting all levels of self, and all of the contracted habits of a lifetime are impacting our current sexual experience. As we work to resolve old patterns of contraction, we will inevitably become aware of sexual memories, choices, issues, and behaviors.

Furthermore, as our breath becomes freer and as we are more consistently resolving past contracted energies, we will find ourselves naturally feeling more sexual. The resolution of the past releases ecstatic energies in the present. Breath is energy moving, which is feelings arising, which, when we utterly encourage emotional freedom, moves easily to sexual excitement: to breathe fully and freely is to be powerfully inspired, sensually aroused, and sexually fulfilled as body, mind, and spirit.

This state of unity is a great leap beyond the typical sexual experience. For all its pleasures, its romances, its mysterious attractions, and its procreative function, common sexual practice is only a taste, a mere hint, of what is possible for humans.

Although this taste can be delicious, tantalizing, and often quite satisfying, for most people, sexual experience ranges from frustratingly limited to dangerously dysfunctional. Even worse, the sexual act tends to be addictive—pursued for and expressive of minor and/or destructive values—and thus degenerates into patterns of contraction. With the passing of time, our sexual experience becomes less conscious and more driven, and we find ourselves less and less able to influence our manner of sexual expression. And as our sexual practices become compulsive habits, we lose the freedom to sense and encourage and, thus, thoroughly embody a dimension of ourselves that is both holy spirit and happy flesh.

Sex is the *feeling* of relationship: it is the sum of our sensory experience and emotional awareness of another living being.

Sexual energy is the energy that connects us to some other—a radiant field emanating out into contact with our world. We are having a sexual experience any time we are feeling a movement toward greater wholeness with some other part of our world. We are healthy sexual creatures to the extent that we desire closer and more intimate contact with another being, or many other beings, or all beings.

Sexual energy is the raw material of our creative efforts. The poet rapturing over the color and smell of a flower is having a peak sexual experience, as may any artist, musician, craftsperson, or performer when they are at their most creative expression. There is strong sexual energy flowing through our money markets and athletic contests, a palpable "juice" that players learn to thrive on. There is shared sexual energy flowing throughout our social affairs and the most violent of sexual energy in our endless wars. And there is a soft, nurturing sexual energy forever passing between parent and child, and kissing cousins, and platonic friends.

All living things are related, and everything is alive. We are connected to all living things through radiant energy fields, and any field grows stronger the more frequent or intimate or "charged" the relationship. Sex is our awareness of the connecting energies; it is a feeling measure of our connectedness to the living things in our world. We grow stronger sexually the more we affirm and celebrate our co-creative relationship with others. And radiating free energy—simple love—is the best of sex, an active blessing for all our relations.

We must at least assume the possibility of living our entire lives in such a state: that we could be vitally whole and sexually thriving individuals; that we could be ever-expanding, as energy, into connectedness with all living things; that we could feel, and thoroughly enjoy, intimate connection with all others; and that we could experience an orgasmic and wondrously creative movement of living energy through loving relationship with any other human, with an animal, with a tree, with a mountain, or with an entire planet. Such is the promise of and for humanity, if our wisest teachers and most advanced sages are to be believed and if, indeed, the song of our hearts is to be heard. How, then, can our actual experience of sexuality be so painfully different?

An old-growth forest can teach us much about sex. It is a lush, teeming profusion of living things and decaying matter, a myriad of comings and goings and birthings and dyings, all interrelated, all interconnected through currents of vital energy that is fervently intercoursing. Every living thing is making love with every other living thing; affect a single relationship and you affect all of the relationships. An old-growth forest is *great sex*—an intricately interwoven and perfectly balanced body of life and death, and left to itself it may go on creating new life forever.

It is instructive that modern industrial culture calls such forests "decadent" and prefers to replace them with straight and sanitary rows of "mono-trees," distinguished by their narrow range of relationship and their sole productive purpose. Modern tree farms show poor resistance to disease and pestilence, fail to hold the soil together, and offer little to the greater family of life. They suffer from an awful sex life and are thus a dying race.

Likewise, the sexual lives of modern men and women are uniformly restricted—and at terrible cost. While delighting in two particular areas of sexual experience—genital play and

procreation—we have lost touch with a universe of loving partners. We have confined our capacity for sexual feelings along
such a narrow spectrum that we are chronically under-
nourished. Even when the sex is good and it flows with the warm-
est of love, we tend to focus on a single partner, a single orgasm,
and the sole purposes of release and procreation.

Like any "mono-crop," we too are showing weakening resistance to disease and pestilence; our shared creative lifestream is
seriously infected. We are limiting our felt, sexual awareness to
but a few of our relations, while contracting from everything
else. We treasure our occasional orgasms as if they were rare and
fleeting gifts, while an ocean of living energies await our loving
and, thus, arousing touch.

It seems a necessary stage in human development that we
separate in this way, that we feel disconnected from other
humans and from the natural environment, and that we have
little experience of joyous and intimate connection with others.
Our promise may be for ecstatic wholeness, but our inherited
reality is painful alienation. Our lives become the drama of
resolving this conflict—we are always yearning for and moving
toward greater wholeness—exploring the issues of relationship
while facing the consequences of living as if we were disconnected, separate, and alone.

Sex is the physical and emotional feeling of this human
drama. "Good sex" is any moment in which we are coming
closer to another—*any other*—and "bad sex" is any moment in
which we are contracting inward and away from more intimate
relationship. Not surprisingly, our primary patterns for sexual
experience—radiating outward as love or contracting inward,
afraid—are formed in our first few minutes, days, and years of life.

Just as we make the mistake of thinking that infants are not conscious, so, despite ample evidence to the contrary, it is generally believed that infants and growing children are not sexual or are presexual. The child's sexual experience is denied, ignored, and avoided until puberty (when, for too many adolescents, it is further denied, ignored, and avoided). It is thought that sex comes with the coming of age and that at the magical point of puberty, sexuality suddenly arises as a new fact of life.

In fact, puberty only confers the ability to procreate through sex—an extraordinary new stage in life, without question. But sexual feeling and the possibility for sexual arousal and expression are fundamental conditions of life prior to puberty, continuing on through old age. We are sexual beings from the very beginning, and our failure to see this and to treat children accordingly is the beginning of all sexual frustration and dysfunction.

Newborns are both hyperconscious and hypersexual, one continuous erogenous zone, from head to toe and inside and out. They are all energy and very little mass (highly advantageous for good sex). They connect urgently and intimately with all local energy fields, with all their relations, with every living thing, with every movement and touch. And all such experience is sexual to them—they feel, they thrill, they open wider and reach deeper. Like the tiniest bird in an old-growth forest, newborns are making love to all of life and creating their own growing lives in the process.

Infants are, however, most fragile lovers and easily wounded, and we must give the greatest of care to the world we provide. Mostly, nothing more is needed than a safe and nourishing environment and the omnipresence of motherlove. It is that simple. As children grow, their field of influence also grows, and we must broaden our support, continuing to provide steady safety and unconditional love as they contact more and more of the world.

Children will energetically embrace *every* living thing they meet—touching it, tasting it, feeling it, testing it, *making love to it.* This world is ever a tingling delight, and with each new day they reach out for more and more of it. If met with peace and nurturance, with love and support, with tender caring, like any lover—*like the most precious lover*—then they will continue to open and expand, growing eagerly into greater and greater connection with the world.

All of our love and support serves in that it allows children to stay open and expanding as creative/sexual/loving energy. Early lessons then affirm the certain good of giving and receiving love, and the safety and pleasure of being energetically connected to others. And, so important, children learn that the body is absolutely the most wonderful thing in the world, an infinite source of beauty and joy.

Such children will grow strong and secure in self-love, since their experience has consistently confirmed their ability to *be love.* Such children may never lose early fairy friends, may never have to leave behind the high-energy reality that comes so naturally to children, yet seems so foreign to adults. Such children will mature sexually as they grow, their bodies and minds moving gracefully forward in balance. Finally, such a childhood is the birthright of every new babe and the surest hope for our planet's future.

Obviously, such a childhood is an ideal, and we cannot hope to spare our children every hurt and disappointment. Still, we must understand that every time a child is met with anger or hate or physical abuse, that child will contract painfully into him or herself, withdrawing from energetic contact with the environment. Every such contraction diminishes the child unless he or she is taught and encouraged to heal and to energetically expand toward wholeness again. All traumas that remain unresolved are carried forward as energetic tension—the mental, physical and emotional patterns that will adversely define the child's life to come.

For every painful event and every pattern of contraction there is a specific manner of breathing, the actual way in which the energetic contraction was embodied. Fortunately, we can teach our children to breathe in new ways, using the breath to loosen and resolve the harshest of pains. And we can breathe deeply and freely for ourselves—for our own inner children—releasing the past and radiating happy love unto all our relations.

Have you ever thought to wonder to yourself what orgasm is? I'll bet you never said to yourself, "Why, it's a spontaneous, reflexive re-distribution of energy." At least I hope not. But orgasm *is* a spontaneous, reflexive re-distribution of energy; and, *because* it is, orgasm is not limited to genital release, nor to sexual contact as a stimulus. It means that sneezes can be orgasmic. It means that the tension you collect between your shoulder blades can release orgasmically. It means that, whenever you have extra energy collected somewhere and you're willing to simply surrender to the tendency of that energy to *move*, you can allow yourself orgasm.

Julie Henderson[26]

Breathing in and out deeply
  through your mouth,
    with the jaw hanging loosely open, and
     your breathing deep, slow, calm, and gentle,
      even as you read
      become aware of the lunar point,
      simple awareness of the lunar point,
   with each slow, gentle breath.
And now with each inhale
  tense the muscles of the lunar point,
   pulling inward and upward,
    inhaling and tightening,
     and now with each exhale
      release the muscles of the lunar point,
      letting go and relaxing,
   exhaling and releasing.
For the next few minutes, continue this
  breathing deep and slow through the mouth,
    tensing the muscles of the lunar point,
    with each gentle inhale,
     pulling inward and upward,
     and releasing all tension
      with each gentle exhale,
      paying attention to the lunar point,
     focused at the lunar point,
  as your eyes gently close . . .

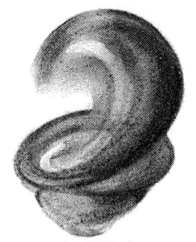

✳ XIII ✳

Sexual Communion

The lower region of the human body (including the sacrum, anus, perineum, genitals, and lower abdomen) is the source and cauldron of extraordinary quantities of sexual energy. This energy is a natural function of physical existence; it arises directly from the cellular structure of the body and is stored as dense, nearly material energy in the bodily "basement" until drawn upon for creative purposes.

For the most part, our sexual energy remains dormant, unfelt, untapped, and unexpressed. Even those with fairly active sexual and creative lives are moving only a small fraction of the energy that all humans carry as latent creative potential. It is rather as if we were going through life with our own private nuclear reactors—tucked away, out of sight, unused, and forgotten.

In the yogic tradition, this latent sexual energy is called *kun-*

dalini, and it is described as a coiled snake resting poised at the base of the spine until the individual, through conscious practice, causes it to awaken and flow upward through the spine. The yogis see kundalini as the energy of human evolution and enlightenment; they also recognize that it is such a powerful force that when prematurely awakened in one who is not ready, rising kundalini can cause serious difficulties (see appendix B).

It is interesting that the symbol of the Western medical system is the caduceus—a straight staff, with two snakes rising from the bottom and coiling upward to the head—and also that it is the snake in Genesis that brings sexuality into the Garden, thus setting humans out on their evolutionary journey. In fact, the snake appears in most of the creation myths of our world, most always as sexual energy. The universal human challenge is to master the snake by allowing its powerful energy to rise from the genitals up through the higher centers of consciousness. That is, our challenge is not to deny sex or suppress it or merely express it, but to vibrationally raise sexual energy and learn to use it for transformational good.

In the Chinese Taoist tradition, it is taught that in addition to raising sexual energy upward through the spine, one must also encourage the energy to flow down the front of the body, gathering it again in the sexual region and thus completing an internal circle. This insight is important, for it stresses the special human balance between Heaven and Earth. We are bodies ascending toward spirit, even as we are spirits descending into flesh.

The human challenge, then, is to raise conscious awareness toward higher dimensions of spirit, even as we are consciously, and ecstatically, grounding ourselves in the body. Likewise, we must extend our sexual energy out into contact with others, even as we are receiving sexual energies into ourselves. We are at our healthiest when we are circulating energy—internally and within our relationships. And there is no more natural and accessible way for achieving this balance than through circular breathing.

Though any two sincere and like-minded people can be effective breathing partners, the best partners will be those who can freely allow sexual arousal to occur during a session. This does not mean that they are breathing for the specific purpose of genital excitement, or that a session without arousal is somehow deficient, or that any genital play is encouraged. It simply means that generating and feeling strong currents of sexual energy is an inevitable result of deep breathing and an essential aspect of any healthy and creatively fulfilling life.

It is quite common during a circular breathing session for one or both of the partners to feel sexually aroused. Often, the two partners will feel arousal simultaneously, even though they are neither touching nor verbally communicating. Such moments of arousal are clear indications that energy is moving throughout each body and that the relationship between the two breathers is safe enough to allow deep and transformational communion.

Of paramount importance is the way in which each of the partners responds to any feelings of arousal. There are historically only two options open for most people: suppress it or express it. We either feel the energy and reactively suppress it by contracting in and away from the external stimulus (that is, another human being), or we feel the energy and rush toward expressing it through genital orgasm.

Suppression, of course, runs counter to the whole purpose of circular breathing and thus only serves to frustrate the process. When the breathing partner suppresses sexual arousal, it leads either to painful intensity, as when the muscles tightly contract (the pain of holding in strong currents of sexual energy), or to phasing out and avoiding the interpersonal contact altogether.

The sitter faces similar problems when suppressing sexual arousal during a breathing session. Boredom, distraction, discomfort, impatience, fatigue—such are the common afflictions of a sexually suppressing sitter, who will have an increasingly difficult time staying alert, focused, and committed to the process.

Expression of sexual arousal through genital orgasm also runs counter to the purpose of circular breathing, which is to feel and allow the free movement of energy *beyond expression.* Though we cannot rule out the possibility of two breathers moving positively toward genital play and expression (especially if they are currently in a physically intimate relationship), for the most part sexual expression during a breathing session is a violation of trust and can lead only to individual contraction and painful difficulties in the relationship.

Viewed within the context of life energy, expression is a missed opportunity; it is settling for a cup of water when an ocean is available. Conscious circular breathing stimulates powerful flows of energy moving throughout the body and beyond, carrying the breather to a state of deep rapture. Discharging the energy through genital release effectively halts the process and greatly limits a breather's capacity for rapture. Thus, even when two breathers can move freely to genital orgasm, there is serious question as to whether it is the best use of their energy.

Each of the partners must be committed to overcoming the patterned reactions of suppression and expression, while staying with the breath and allowing the feelings of energy to radiate throughout and beyond the body. Suppression is overcome by continuing to breathe while enjoying the sensations of energetic excitement; expression is overcome by continuing to breathe while extending conscious awareness to nongenital areas of the body and beyond.

This is not intended as a blanket condemnation of suppression and expression as life options. There may always be cultural and social situations during which the individual suppression of sexual energy is the optimal thing to do. However, engineering such suppression as a conscious choice—with full attention to energetic consequences—is quite different from going through life with an unconscious pattern of contraction that is negatively directing and impeding the flow of one's energy.

Likewise, the expression of sexual energy through genital play and orgasm is vital for the procreation of new life and every bit as vital as a simple, and healing, human pleasure. But, again, expressing sexual energy as a conscious and deliberate choice— with full attention to energetic consequences—is hardly a description of common sexual practices. Indeed, few people are aware of sexual fulfillment that does not *of necessity* involve genital play and orgasm; we are not even led to expect other choices.

We have seriously missed the serpent's message and promise. It is in moving sexual energy *throughout* the body that our deepest rapture arises; it is in *extending* our most precious feelings of rapture to another that the holy blessing of sexual communion is given/received.

We can never realize such communion with another if we always follow the demands of our genitals. Like a siren call, genital orgasm pulls us to the brink of deep communion, only to leave us suddenly exhausted and feeling oddly separate. Nor will suppression ever bring us anything but frustration, contraction, and further suppression. Somehow, we must stop saying no to sex, while at the same time finding a whole new way to say yes.

To return to our breathing partners. . .[27] They are breathing, their energies are moving, it is feeling good, exciting, even sexually arousing, and then. . . what? The answer, it should not be surprising, is to *feel and breathe*. The breathers must remain committed to full awareness of all arising feelings, while continuing to breathe and encouraging the free circulation of energy. That the arising feelings are sexual and the genitals are becoming aroused is all the more reason for full feeling awareness and the affirmation of breath.

It is so important that the breathers *enjoy* any sexual feelings—that they allow the feelings to be joyful. If a breather's immediate reaction to sexual arousal is "Oh no, I mustn't" or "Oh no, this is bad," then the event is already contracting toward suppression or dysfunctional expression. Sexual energy arising in the body is a most delicious offering; the breathers must open to it, receive it, love it, and thoroughly enjoy it.

At the same time, all arising energies/feelings must be allowed and encouraged to move. Specifically, sexual energy, as it arises in the genitals, must be circulated throughout the body and beyond. To achieve this, the breather first can inhale while drawing energy up the spine, thus establishing flow away from the genitals. Continuing, the breather can inhale, drawing the energy from the lower spine to the heart, and then exhale, while radiating energy, as love, to the partner.

Inhaling, the energy is consciously drawn into free circulation; exhaling, the energy is released and extended as love. It rarely takes more than a few minutes of such conscious circular breathing to move a breather from genital fixation to an all-over tingling feeling of rapture.

This is the full practice of circular breathing: always breathing and always saying yes to all arising feelings. When energy becomes strongly focused in any one place—and especially in the genital region—then the breather consciously uses the breath to circulate the energy, drawing it to the heart, where it is radiated out as love. In its fullest, this is an alchemy of the heart—the transmutation of energy into flesh and the infusion of flesh with living, loving spirit.

As this practice continues, each partner (or lover) is committed to breathing, generating and circulating great flows of energy, sustaining joyful awareness of all feelings, and radiating, as conscious love, into connection with the other. This engenders the experience of sexual communion—two living creatures joyfully sharing breath/energy/feeling/love with each other. The most intimate and profoundly creative of experiences, sexual communion is nonetheless as simple as breath for those who have learned to simply breathe.

It is most important that we learn to practice Full Awareness of Breathing during our daily lives. Usually, when we perform our tasks, our thoughts wander, and our joys, sorrows, anger, and unease follow close behind. Although we are alive, we are not able to bring our minds into the present moment, and we live in forgetfulness.

We can begin by becoming aware of our breath, by following our breathing. Breathing in and breathing out, we know we are breathing in and out, and we can smile to affirm that we are ourselves, that we are in control of ourselves. Through awareness of breathing, we can be awake in and to the present moment.

Thich Nhat Hanh[28]

Pay attention to your next few breaths.
Even as you continue to read these words,
  also notice that you are breathing,
    and that it is easy to read and to breathe
    and to be aware of breath,
    all in the same moment.
Pay attention to the quality of each inhale.
Even as you read, notice the feelings and
  sensations of energy flowing into your body.
Feel the places in your torso that move
  or do not move with each inhalation.
Pay attention to the quality of each exhale.
Even as you read, notice the feelings and
  sensations of energy flowing from your body.
Feel the places in your torso that move or
  do not move with each exhalation.
Now return to the top of this page
  and read through again,
    paying close attention
    to the ebb and flow of each breath,
      even as you are paying close attention
      to the sound and meaning of each word,
      and for a minute or so,
      simply pay attention to yourself breathing,
as your eyes softly close . . .

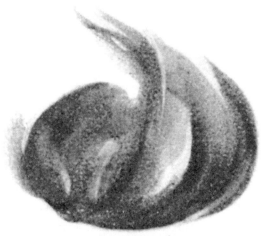

✳ XIV ✳

The Holy Breath

The primary and essential function of breath is reception and release. With each inhale, we open to, draw in, conduct, and thus receive the living, spiritual energies of the universe. With each exhale, we surrender, relax, radiate as love, and thus release all personal energies into universal relationship.

Every such breath is a drink from God's own fountain and will provide the fundamental nourishment that humans require. Every such breath is a conscious movement of pleasure—throughout all levels of self—richly felt and deeply healing. And, truly, every such breath is *deserved*: we are children of breath, and the way is ever open for our return to a life divine and everlasting.

With time, we may notice that our way of breathing perfectly reflects our way of life. The saying, "As we live and breathe. . ." is precisely true: we breathe to live, of course, and we live in the manner that we breathe.

The inhale relates to will. It is the embodiment of intention, drive, desire, wanting, and receiving. When there is a tired, negligible, or complacent inhale (typically leading to phasing out), it reflects similar attitudes toward life: "I can't, I don't want to, it's too much effort, it'll never work, I don't deserve it."

When there is a vital, urgent thirsting for each breath (typically leading to intensity), it reflects a strong, inherent desire for life: the breather is inspired, and inspiring, and is gathering in the requisite energies of a creative life.

Attention also must be given to the physical movement of each inhale. To live fully is to breathe in fully—to move and fill the whole torso with breath/energy. To breathe only into the upper chest is to avoid the strong, creative energies of the lower abdomen and sexual organs. To breathe only into the belly is to avoid the equally strong, creative energies of the heart and throat.

Through observation of the inhale, we can see those areas of experience that the breather would avoid—areas where the breather's will is inhibited. Conversely, through consciously bringing the breath into such areas, the will is exercised and strengthened, and inhibiting patterns of contraction are finally resolved.

The exhale relates to surrender. It is the embodiment of letting go, relaxing, going with the flow, and releasing. The perfect exhale is completely effortless—it is, precisely, the cessation of all effort, of all doing, of all controlling. At the fullness of the inhale, all doing ceases; the breather surrenders, and the body exhales freely and completely.

Any effort added to the exhale effectively contracts the breather's energy. When, for instance, the breather holds the breath back, letting it out only slowly or not emptying out completely (typically leading to phasing out), the tension of that effort derives from and contributes to patterns of contraction. Such restrained and/or partial exhaling reflects a fundamental distrust toward life, perhaps a belief that there is not enough, and always a belief in the need to stay in control of events.

The breather might also add effort to the exhale by forcefully blowing the air out (typically leading to intensity). Rather than releasing the breath, the breather is urgently pushing it away. Such exhaling reflects a belief that we are filled with "bad" energies, pains, thoughts, and feelings, and that if we work hard enough we can expel/purge them from our system.

It is important to remember that our patterns of contraction, and all possible manifestations of such patterns, are forever comprised of energy—the energy of life itself. *It is not the energy that is bad or unhealthy; rather, it is our choice to hold onto and contract it that is detrimental for us.*

That is, at some time in the past we were in the midst of a challenging event, with energy generating within us to meet the challenge, and *we chose* to contract. It is sustaining that choice now that hurts—not the "old" energy. And strenuously trying to rid oneself of "old" energy (trying to dump the garbage) only serves to add to contraction—is in fact a reflection of the original choice—while directly reinforcing the notion that the breather is inherently unhealthy. In the moment that we resolve such a choice, the long-contracted energy is released and experienced as joy. Indeed, resolving an old pattern is a gift of living, creative energy to the breather and to the surrounding environment.

To repeat, any effort added to the exhale effectively contracts the breather's energy—actually derives from and adds to the breather's patterns of contractions. When we add effort to the exhale, we are creating hardship by working where no work is required and by struggling unnecessarily with a fundamentally free process of life.

Furthermore, as the exhale becomes stuck and inhibited, it becomes harder and harder to inhale fully. The less empty we become in breathing out, the less we can hope to fully breathe in anew. The more we hang onto the "stuff" of the past, the more we restrict our present and future potential. Indeed, most problems with an inhibited will/inhale actually begin as problems with surrendering/exhaling. Thus, we should always pay close attention to the exhale and to any feelings and sensations of added effort.

Ultimately, a healthy, balanced, and creative life is comprised of equal parts of will and surrender. We are the doer, exerting our personal will, *and* life is done magically through us, the more we let go. We create the world *and* we surrender to its creations. We are going with the flow down life's river *and* we have the paddle of personal will to steer the way.

When there is too much personal will and not enough surrender or too much surrendering and a weak will, then life is unbalanced and creativity suffers. Such imbalance is always reflected in breath as an imbalance between inhalation/reception and exhalation/release. Conversely, by simply bringing consciousness to the breath—inhaling deeply and fully releasing the exhale—we can actively create resolution and balance, strengthening our personal will while greatly enhancing our capacity for surrender.

Still, as we have seen, we may struggle so with simply breathing—with simply receiving and simply releasing. Old patterns of contraction interfere and impede. Our lungs are filled with the dust of the past; we seem unable to get enough air, we seem unable to really let go. To our great frustration, the more urgently we reach for more breath, the more we notice how little we breathe, and how often we stop breathing, and how easily we just forget the whole thing.

For whatever solace—and encouragement—it may provide, a growing awareness of how hard, and even painful, it is to breathe is actually a sign of progress. Prior to consciously working with the breath, most people have no awareness of their breathing at all, except when it seriously malfunctions. The conscious breather, in feeling and moving toward the full power and promise of the breath, becomes more acutely aware of tendencies to contract the breath that have always been unconsciously supported.

Conscious breathing obviously does not create contracted breathing—it reveals it. Thus, the conscious breather who is lately noticing breathing patterns—*I never breathe when I talk to my mother, I didn't breathe through my entire commute to work, I seem to hold my breath whenever I think hard about something, I never breathe when I think about money, I just can't get a full breath!*—is actually breathing better than ever. The struggle is all a sign of healing, though certainly it is a measure of healing that goes down better with a steady patience and a good sense of humor.

Another aspect of the conscious breather's progress, with which we may also struggle, is a growing sense of vulnerability. Our patterns of contraction have long functioned as a form of protection, a literal suit of armor. That we no longer need the protection and that we are suffocating inside the armor does not seem to matter: we are accustomed to this way—it has worked for many years, and it *feels* safe.

To let go of our patterns of protection is to step out of the armor, naked and open to the world and all that it offers. This can be, to say the least, terrifying. However, we can only know how safe the world truly is, and how much love and support there is for each of us, by facing life *without the armor*. Our ideas about the world, formed from inside the armor, are always skewed, false, and limiting, though invariably self-confirming.

In approaching the world as vulnerable, we create a world that no longer threatens. This requires a leap of faith—many leaps of faith—and the courage to breathe in deeply in the midst of difficult times. When "I breathe it in and surrender!" has replaced "I contract from it" as our immediate response to stressful events, then we have transformed the world and our place within it.

Inhaling and exhaling, receiving and releasing, one continuous flow of life: without holding, without pushing, without contracting, and without effort . . .

Inhaling and exhaling, receiving and releasing, one continuous flow of life: with feeling, with pleasure, and with conscious attention to the ever-rising possibility of joy . . .

Simply breathing—simply choosing to breathe, *now*, with conscious, creative awareness—can be the resolution of all that has come before and the evolution of all to follow.

May your every breath bring you peace and joy.
May all beings breathe free and flourish.

Religions are numberless
sects many
yet all follow only two ways:
one takes you to knowledge
and the other to love.
Reaching the goal
one discovers with surprise
that there is no knowledge
separate from love;
that, truly, love is knowledge
and that the secret gate
to both is one:
the breath.

C.M. Chen[29]

✳ APPENDIX A ✳
Conscious Breathing Patterns

There is no right way to breathe at all times. Rather, a conscious breather, through continuously resolving patterns of contraction, will come to breathe spontaneously and effectively according to the demands of a specific situation.

As a general rule, breathing through the nose tends to be more calming and centering, while breathing through the mouth tends to be more exciting and expansive.

Circular breathing has been described and recommended as one way to resolve patterns of contraction. There are innumerable other breathing practices—some quite different from circular breathing—that have also proven valuable to conscious breathers.

It is suggested that the following processes be read and understood and then practiced as meditations, with eyes closed, while either sitting or reclining.

The Cleansing Breath

Breathing in through the nose, with each inhale imagine, sense, feel, or believe that the air is coming in through the soles of your feet. Breathe in *as if* you have to pull the air up through your feet, ankles, legs, hips, and torso, until you blow it out through your open mouth. Continue for several breaths, drawing the air in through your feet and up through your body, and then blowing it out, slowly and calmly.

Now, continuing with this breath, imagine that as you draw the air up through your body you are sweeping along with it all of the contracted energy in your system. Breathe up through the feet, up through your body, sweeping along all contracted energies, and then blow them out—calmly, slowly—with the air. Feel this movement of air and the sweeping of energy as vividly as you can. Really *feel* it.

Now, imagine that as the swept-up energy hits the open air it bursts into a shower of sparks. Picture this, sense it, imagine that with every slow, calm exhale your swept-up energy bursts into a shower of bright sparks.

Continue for several minutes, observing all reactions and sensations, and then follow with a few minutes of slow circular breathing.

Deep-Release Breathing

Breathe in through the nose, and then breathe out through the mouth. At the end of the exhale, pause—*wait, wait, patiently, consciously wait*—until *the body* initiates the next inhale.

Every breath in, through the nose, is slow and calm. At the top of the inhale, release the air through the open mouth—slowly and calmly—and then, with the mouth open and the jaw relaxed, pause—*patiently and consciously wait*—until the body breathes again.

The key to the pause between breaths is in remaining conscious, focused, and purposefully waiting until the body chooses to inhale. If the mind wanders, the breath will revert to its usual unconscious patterns.

Now, during each pause, allow your body to deeply relax and let go. Let the time between breaths be a time of whole body release. *Feel* your body wonderfully letting go.

Now, breathe *into* a specific body area in need of healing or relaxing, and then consciously let all tension go with the exhale, relaxing even further during the pause.

For several breaths, continue breathing into and then releasing and relaxing a specific body part.

Follow with a few minutes of circular breathing.

Retention Breath

Breathe in through the nose, slowly and calmly, and at the top of the inhale, hold the breath in. Do this without straining or tensing—gently hold the breath in.

For several moments, feel the retained energy circulating and radiating throughout the body. Hold the breath in, without tension, and feel the retained energy moving throughout the body. Let it *feel good*—let it be a feeling of pleasure spreading throughout your body.

When it is time to exhale, release the breath—calmly, slowly—through the mouth, and then pause between breaths, waiting patiently for the next inhale. Continue for several minutes.

Now breathe in through the nose and retain the breath, focusing the held energy in a specific part of the body. Hold easily, without tension, feeling pleasure, until it is time to exhale. Then release the energy, and pause between breaths, relaxing even further.

Continue this exercise for several minutes, and follow with circular breathing.

Rhythmic Breathing

Breathing in a steady, controlled rhythm for a sustained period can have a calming, centering, and energizing effect for the breather. Following are some long-practiced rhythms:

Breathe in through the nose for a slow count of 8, hold for 4 counts, breathe out through the nose for a slow count of 8, and pause for 4 counts. Continue for several minutes.

From the Sufis: Breathe in through the nose for a slow count of 7, hold for 1 beat, and breathe out through the nose for a slow count of 7, pausing for 1 beat. Continue for several minutes.

From the Tibetans: Breathe in through the nose for a slow count of 8, hold for 32 counts, and breathe out through the nose for a slow count of 16. Continue for several minutes, with no pause after the exhale.

Feel free to experiment with rhythms—what matters is settling into a soothing, calming flow. Rhythmic breathing is also great while walking (timed by your steps), running, biking, and most other forms of exercise.

Alternate Nostril Breathing

During the course of a day our breath tends to flow more strongly through one nostril than the other, naturally switching dominance every four hours. This reflects our basic polarities of brain, body, mind, and personality—the breath moving back and forth, helping to sustain balance.

We can assist the breath in its balancing act with conscious alternate nostril breathing:

Place the thumb under one nostril, closing it off, and breathe in for a slow count of 8. Hold for 4 counts, while moving the thumb to the other nostril, and then breathe out for a slow count of 8. Pause for 4 counts. Continue for several minutes, always remembering to switch nostrils just before the exhale.

Circulating Energy

Breathe slowly, in and out through the nose.

As you breathe in, feel that you are drawing the air in through your left hand and up your left arm to the base of your neck.

Breathing out, allow the energy to flow down your right arm and out your right hand and fingers.

Continue for several breaths. Then reverse the flow, inhaling up through your right arm and exhaling down your left arm, for several breaths.

Now switch to your legs, inhaling up your left leg to the base of your spine and exhaling down your right leg, for several breaths, then reversing: up the right leg and down the left leg, for several breaths.

Now start the breath at the base of the spine, inhaling while drawing the energy up to the top of your head and then exhaling, letting the energy flow down across your face, throat, chest, belly, and sexual organs.

Continue for several minutes, circulating the energy up the spine with each inhale and letting it flow—like a waterfall—down the front of your body with each exhale.

Conscious Breathing for Lovers

Those who are sexually intimate can use conscious circular breathing to greatly enhance their relationship. The experience of sexual communion is especially suited for lovers, though they must show discipline in foregoing, or at least postponing, genital orgasm. It is recommended that lovers explore the practice of sexual communion in a gradual manner, allowing for a gentle transformation of their relationship to each other and to their world.

The following practices are particulary effective for lovers:

Sit facing one another, either in chairs or cross-legged, but comfortable enough to be able to sit for a long period without changing positions.

Make eye contact, and without touching, find a gentle breathing rhythm, breathing together, each easily following the other. If there is a break in the eye contact, or if the breathing falls out of sync, or if there is a need for emotional expression, allow these things to happen, always returning easily to the breath. Continue with this breathing for a sustained period.

Lie together in bed, with clothing off, side by side, but not touching. Find a deep circular breathing rhythm, breathing together, each easily following the other.

Pay close attention to the feelings in the body, to all sensations, to all emotions, to all movements of energy. Be especially attentive to any tensions; notice the places in the body that first begin to tense, and release and relax with every exhaled breath. Allow for arousal *and* relaxation.

After a time, allow the slightest of contact between bodies—fingers barely touching, or toes. Continue with the breathing and with the relaxation of all tensions.

Usually, this will lead to lovemaking. As it does, remain very conscious of the breath and of your ability to relax. Go slowly. Continue to breath as one. If you feel yourself losing control— being swept along in a sexual rush—then come apart, relax, and follow the breath for a stretch.

Remember to circulate the energy, to move it from the genitals up and to the heart, and to extend the energy as love to your partner.

Sometimes this practice will lead to genital orgasm and other times to a feeling of profound joy and fulfillment without orgasm. At all times, remember to breathe deeply and enjoy.

✳ APPENDIX B ✳
Kundalini Crisis & Spiritual Emergency

The practice of deep circular breathing encourages strong flows of life energy and the release of long-held psycho-emotional patterns of contraction. At times, an individual's experience as the energy moves can be quite upsetting, and it may elevate into a kundalini crisis, or spiritual emergency—a time of crisis caused by the rapid emergence of a new energetic reality. A wide range of physical, mental, emotional, and spiritual effects may occur, as described throughout this book. At their worst, such effects may resemble psychotic episodes, nervous breakdowns, or severe bouts of depression.

Understood within the context of life energy, all such effects represent a healing in process: the individual is in the midst of resolving deep and significant patterns of contraction. A resolution is unfolding but is not yet complete; thus the individual's present-time experience is of *emergency*, of changes emerging. While this may be easily accepted *during* a breathing session, it is possible that some effects will emerge in between sessions, which can be especially upsetting.

An individual in crisis is first and always reminded to breathe. A simple calming breath, slow and gentle through the nose, following an easy rhythm and sustained for several minutes, will encourage relaxation and peaceful resolution. Also, any form of bodywork or massage therapy that can help one to physically and emotionally relax will be very helpful during a crisis. Likewise, acupuncture tends to balance the body's energies, thus helping in a crisis.

Traditional Western medicine is most emphatically *not* recommended for those in the midst of kundalini crisis, or spiritual emergency. With little or no understanding of energy, and thus the effects of moving energy, it is impossible for Western medical practitioners to understand what is happening during a crisis. Typically, they will diagnose an individual as sick/ill/unhealthy and then prescribe medication, hospitalization, or electroshock therapy. Typically, people do not improve from such treatments, and, tragically, our mental health system is filled with people who were energetically evolving until they landed in a mental health expert's office.

Kundalini crisis is a healing in process; spiritual emergency is a more spiritual self rapidly emerging. We must encourage full resolution by continuing to breathe, following our feelings, physically relaxing in any way possible, and trusting implicitly in the process.

The following two books deal with emerging crises and can be very helpful: *Kundalini: Psychosis or Transcendence*, by Lee Sannella (H.R. Dakin, 1976) and *Spiritual Emergency*, by Stanislav and Christina Grof (Jeremy Tarcher, 1989).

✳ APPENDIX C ✳
The Breath We Share

"Did you know that the average breath you breathe contains about 10 sextillion atoms, a number which, as you may remember, can be written in modern notation as 10^{22}? And, since the entire atmosphere of Earth is voluminous enough to hold about the same number of breaths, each breath turns out, like man himself, to be about midway in size between an atom and the world—mathematically speaking, 10^{22} atoms in each of the 10^{22} breaths multiplying to a total of 10^{44} atoms of air blowing around the planet. This means of course that each time you inhale you are drawing into yourself an average of about one atom from each of the breaths contained in the whole sky. Also every time you exhale you are sending back the same average of an atom to each of these breaths, as is every other living person, and this exchange, repeated twenty thousand times a day by some four billion people, has the surprising consequence that each breath you breathe must contain a quadrillion (10^{15}) atoms breathed by the rest of mankind within the past few weeks and more than a million atoms breathed personally sometime by each and any person on Earth. . . .

"With such information you can more easily accept the fact that your next breath will include a million odd atoms of oxygen and nitrogen once breathed by Pythagoras, Socrates, Confucius, Moses, Columbus, Einstein or anyone you can think of, including a lot from the Chinese in China within a fortnight, from bushmen in South Africa, Eskimos in Greenland. . . And, going on to animals, you may add a few million molecules from the mighty blowings of the whale that swallowed Jonah, from the snorts of Muhammad's white mare, from the restive raven that Noah sent forth from the ark. Then to the vegetable king-dom, including exhalations from the bo tree under which Bud-dha heard the Word of God, from the ancient cycads bent by wallowing dinosaurs in 150 million B.C. And don't forget swamps themselves and the ancient seas where atoms are liquid and more numerous, and the solid Earth where they are more numerous still, the gases, liquids and solids in these mediums all circulating their atoms and molecules at their natural rates, interchanging, evaporating, condensing and diffusing them in a complex global metabolism."

Guy Murchie[30]

Notes

1. Walt Whitman, "Passage To India," in *Leaves of Grass* (New York: The New American Library of World Literature, Inc., 1954), 328.

2. Da Free John, *The Eating Gorilla Comes in Peace* (Clearlake: The Dawn Horse Press, 1979), 298.

3. Sondra Ray, *Celebration of Breath* (Berkeley: Celestial Arts, 1983), 37.

4. Pundit Acharya, *Breath, Sleep, the Heart, and Life* (Clearlake, CA: The Dawn Horse Press, 1975), 177.

5. Energy in living systems must be thought of as particle/wave. As particle, energy flows; as wave, it radiates.

6. Frederick Leboyer, *Birth Without Violence* (New York: Alfred A. Knopf, 1976), 109.

7. Da Free John, *Conscious Exercise and the Transcendental Sun* (Clearlake, CA: The Dawn Horse Press, 1977), 216-17.

8. Thich Nhat Hanh, *The Sutra on the Full Awareness of Breathing* (Berkeley: Parallax Press, 1988), 53.

9. Julie Henderson, *The Lover Within* (Barrytown, NY: Station Hill, 1986), 25.

10. Whitman, "There Was a Child Went Forth," in *Leaves of Grass*, 290.

11. The reader is referred to Thomas Verny, *The Secret Life of the Unborn Child* (New York: Summit Books, 1983); Michael Odent, *Birth Reborn* (New York: Random House, 1988); David Chamberlain, *Babies Remember Birth* (Los Angeles: Jeremy Tarcher, 1988).

12. Leboyer, *Birth Without Violence*, 51.

13. The reader is referred to Jeanne Achterberg, *Imagery in Healing, Shamanism and Modern Medicine* (Boston: Shambhala, 1985); and B. Ehrenreich and D. English, *Witches, Midwives, and Nurses: A History of Women Healers* (New York: The Feminist Press, 1973).

14. Bruno Hans Geba, *Breathe Away Your Tension* (New York: Random House, 1973), 38.

15. Tarthang Tulku, *Gesture of Balance* (Emeryville, CA: Dharma Publishing, 1977), 65.

16. Stanislav Grof, *The Adventure of Self-Discovery* (Albany: State University of New York Press, 1988), 170.

17. There are many different approaches to hyperventilation. Circular breathing is strongly recommended because of its simplicity and its inherent safety.

18. Grof, *Adventure of Self-Discovery*, 171.

19. Ray, *Celebration of Breath*, 5.

20. Those with heart problems, internal bleeding, or epilepsy and women in the advanced stages of pregnancy should approach circular breathing with gentle caution. Each of these conditions can be helped with deep breathing as long as the individual works slowly, patiently, and with a healthy respect for the body's present limitations. *See* appendix B.

21. Stanislav and Christina Grof have made extensive use of music during breathing sessions, and provide a complete explanation and iconography in their book *The Adventure of Self-Discovery* (Albany: State University of New York Press, 1988.)

22. Ray, *Celebration of Breath*, 40.

23. Tarthang Tulku, *Kum Nye Relaxation* (Berkeley: Dharma Publishing, 1978), 42.

24. Pundit Acharya, *Breath, Sleep, the Heart, and Life*, 129.

25. Da Free John, *Love of the Two Armed Form* (Clearlake, CA: The Dawn Horse Press, 1978), 249.

26. Henderson, *The Lover Within*, 85.

27. Everything that will be said about the process of circulating energy between breathing partners can be applied to virtually any human relationship. This discussion is *especially* germane to the parent-child relationship and the feelings of sexual arousal that so often occur between parent and child.

28. Thich Nhat Hanh, *Sutra on the Full Awareness of Breathing*, 44.

29. Frederick Leboyer, *The Art of Breathing* (London: Element Books, 1979), 1.

30. Guy Murchie, *The Seven Mysteries of Life* (Boston: Houghton Mifflin Co., 1981), 320-321.

Permissions

Special thanks to Kösel-Verlag for permission to reprint the C.M. Chen poem from *Die Kunst zu Atman* by Frederick Leboyer, copyright © Kösel-Verlag, München; copyright © for the English translation of the poem: Element Books. Thanks also to Houghton Mifflin Co. for permission to reprint excerpts from *The Seven Mysteries of Life*, copyright © 1978 by Guy Murchie.

About the Author

Michael Sky is a holistic healer and firewalking instructor. Since 1976, he has maintained a private practice as a rebirther and polarity therapist focusing on breath, life energy, and the positive benefits of deep relaxation. He travels widely, leading workshops in the exploration of breathing, firewalking, bodywork, and the effective use of ritual.

Michael has facilitated firewalking workshops for more than three thousand people since 1984. He is the author of *Dancing with the Fire* (Bear & Company, 1989), a comprehensive exploration of the scientific, psychological, and spiritual teachings of fire. Michael has also produced a video documenting the ancient ritual of the firewalk. He and his wife, Penny Sharp, publish the nationally distributed environmental newsletter *Dragonfly Quarterly* and are residents of Orcas Island, Washington.

To write to the author:

Michael Sky
P. O. Box 1085
Eastsound, WA 98245